DISABILITY STUDIES

PARKINSON'S DISEASE

AWARENESS AMONG YOUNG ADULTS

Disability Studies

Joav Merrick - Series Editor -

Medical Director, Ministry of Social Affairs,
Jerusalem, Israel

**Parkinson's Disease:
Awareness among Young Adults**
Ronald Chow, Jaclyn Viehweger, Michael Borean, Drew Hollenberg, and Joav Merrick (Editors)
2017. ISBN: 978-1-53612-745-4 (Hardcover)
2018. ISBN: 978-1-53612-745-4 (Softcover)
2017. ISBN: 978-1-53612-746-1 (e-book)

**Human Development:
Equipping Minds with Cognitive Development**
Carol T. Brown and Joav Merrick
2018. ISBN: 978-1-53613-053-9 (Softcover)
2018. ISBN: 978-1-53613-054-6 (e-book)

**Autism Spectrum Disorder:
Awareness among Young Adults**
Ronald Chow, Jaclyn Viehweger, Joav Merrick (Editors)
2017. ISBN: 978-1-53612-730-0 (Hardcover)
2017. ISBN: 978-1-53612-731-7 (e-book)

**Virtual Reality:
Recent Advances in Virtual Rehabilitation System Design**
Wendy Powell, Albert "Skip" Rizzo, Paul M. Sharkey and Joav Merrick
2017. ISBN: 978-1-53612-040-0 (Softcover)
2017. ISBN: 978-1-53612-061-5 (e-book)

**Child Abuse:
Children with Disabilities**
Vincent J Palusci, Dena Nazer, Donald E Greydanus and Joav Merrick
2017. ISBN: 978-1-53612-035-6 (Hardcover)
2017. ISBN: 978-1-53612-056-1 (e-book)

Rehabilitation: Innovations and Challenges in the Use of Virtual Reality Technologies
Wendy Powell, Albert "Skip" Rizzo, Paul M. Sharkey and Joav Merrick, (Editors)
2017. ISBN: 978-1-53612-080-6 (Hardcover)
2017. ISBN: 978-1-53612-099-8 (e-book)

Virtual Reality: Recent Advances for Health and Wellbeing
Wendy Powell, Paul M Sharkey and Albert "Skip" Rizzo
2017. ISBN: 978-1-53612-454-5 (Softcover)
2017. ISBN: 978-1-53612-455-2 (e-book)

Pediatric Pain: Current Aspects
Hatim A. Omar, Dilip R. Patel, Donald E. Greydanus, and Joav Merrick (Editors)
2016. ISBN: 978-1-63485-505-1 (Hardcover)
2016. ISBN: 978-1-63485-537-2 (e-book)

Recent Advances on Using Virtual Reality Technologies for Rehabilitation
Paul M. Sharkey and Joav Merrick (Editors)
2016. ISBN: 978-1-63484-027-9 (Hardcover)
2015. ISBN: 978-1-63484-028-6 (e-book)

Technology, Rehabilitation and Empowerment of People with Special Needs
Lena Pareto, Paul M Sharkey and Joav Merrick (Editors)
2015. ISBN: 978-1-63482-713-3 (Hardcover)
2015. ISBN: 978-1-63482-737-9 (e-book)

Virtual Reality: Rehabilitation in Motor, Cognitive and Sensorial Disorders
Paul M. Sharkey and Joav Merrick (Editors)
2014. ISBN: 978-1-63321-773-7 (Hardcover)
2014. ISBN: 978-1-63321-787-4 (e-book)

Virtual Reality: People with Special Needs
Paul M. Sharkey and Joav Merrick (Editors)
2014. ISBN: 978-1-63321-729-4 (Hardcover)
2014. ISBN: 978-1-63321-734-8 (e-book)

Quality of Life and Intellectual Disability: Knowledge Application to other Social and Educational Challenges
Roy I. Brown and Rhonda M. Faragher (Editors)
2014. ISBN: 978-1-62948-264-4 (Hardcover)
2014. ISBN: 978-1-62948-272-9 (e-book)

Intellectual Disability: Some Current Issues
Joav Merrick, Donald E Greydanus and Dilip R. Patel (Editors)
2014. ISBN: 978-1-63321-855-0 (Hardcover)
2014. ISBN: 978-1-63321-867-3 (e-book)

From One Century to the Next: A History of Wrentham State School and the Institutional Model in Massachusetts
Ingrid Grenon
2014. ISBN: 978-1-63117-711-8 (Hardcover)
2014. ISBN: 978-1-63483-805-4 (Softcover)
2014. ISBN: 978-1-63117-712-5 (e-book)

Pain and the Elderly
Joav Merrick and Mimi M.Y. Tse
2013. ISBN: 978-1-62948-468-6 (Hardcover)
2013. ISBN: 978-1-62948-475-4 (e-book)

Pain: International Research in Pain Management
Joav Merrick, Patricia Schofield and Mohammed Morad (Editors)
2013. ISBN: 978-1-62948-423-5 (Hardcover)
2013. ISBN: 978-1-62948-435-8 (e-book)

Disability and Chronic Disease
Joav Merrick, Shoshana Aspler and Mohammed Morad (Editors)
2013. ISBN: 978-1-62948-288-0 (Hardcover)
2013. ISBN: 978-1-62948-307-8 (e-book)

Down Syndrome and Dementia. A Comprehensive and Historical Review
Vee P. Prasher
2012. ISBN: 978-1-62081-263-1 (Hardcover)
2012. ISBN: 978-1-62081-271-6 (e-book)

Rett Syndrome: Therapeutic Interventions
Meir Lotan and Joav Merrick (Editors)
2011. ISBN: 978-1-61728-614-8 (Hardcover)
2011. ISBN: 978-1-61728-080-1 (Softcover)
2011. ISBN: 978-1-61761-131-5 (e-book)

Pain Management Yearbook 2010
Joav Merrick (Editor)
2011. ISBN: 978-1-61209-972-9 (Hardcover)
2011. ISBN: 978-1-62808-255-5 (e-book)

Pain Management Yearbook 2009
Joav Merrick (Editor)
2011. ISBN: 978-1-61209-666-7 (Hardcover)
2011. ISBN: 978-1-62081-774-2 (e-book)

Pain. Brain Stimulation in the Treatment of Pain
Helena Knotkova, Ricardo Cruciani and Joav Merrick (Editors)
2011. ISBN: 978-1-60876-690-1 (Hardcover)
2011. ISBN: 978-1-61470-495-9 (e-book)

Neural Plasticity in Chronic Pain
Helena Knotkova, Ricardo A. Cruciani and Joav Merrick (Editors)
2011. ISBN: 978-1-61324-657-3 (Hardcover)
2011. ISBN: 978-1-62417-407-0 (e-book)

Disability from a Humanistic Perspective: Towards a Better Quality of Life
Shunit Reiter
2011. ISBN: 978-1-60456-412-9 (Hardcover)
2011. ISBN: 978-1-63117-654-8 (e-book)

Cancer in Children and Adults with Intellectual Disabilities: Current Research Aspects
Daniel Satgé and Joav Merrick (Editors)
2011. ISBN: 978-1-61761-856-7 (Hardcover)
2011. ISBN: 978-1-61122-187-9 (e-book)

Contemporary Issues in Intellectual Disabilities
V. P. Prasher
2010. ISBN: 978-1-61668-023-7 (Hardcover)
2010. ISBN: 978-1-61209-292-8 (e-book)

DISABILITY STUDIES

PARKINSON'S DISEASE

AWARENESS AMONG YOUNG ADULTS

RONALD CHOW
JACLYN VIEHWEGER
MICHAEL BOREAN
DREW HOLLENBERG
AND
JOAV MERRICK
EDITORS

nova biomedical
New York

Library of Congress Cataloging-in-Publication Data

ISBN: 978-1-53612-745-4
Library of Congress Control Number: 2017957257

Published by Nova Science Publishers, Inc. † New York

CONTENTS

INTRODUCTION

In: Parkinson's Disease
Editors: Ronald Chow, et al.
ISBN: 978-1-53612-745-4

Chapter 1

HOW AWARE/KNOWLEDGEABLE ARE YOUNG ADULTS ABOUT PARKINSON'S DISEASE?

Ronald Chow[1,*], BMSc(C), Michael Borean[1], BMSc(C), Drew Hollenberg[1], BMSc(C) and Joav Merrick[2-6], MD, MMedSc, DMSc

[1]Infinitas Research Group, London, Ontario, Canada,
[2]National Institute of Child Health and Human Development, Jerusalem, Israel,
[3]Office of the Medical Director, Health Services, Division for Intellectual and Developmental Disabilities, Ministry of Social Affairs and Social Services, Jerusalem, Israel,
[4]Division of Pediatrics, Hadassah Hebrew University Medical Centre, Mt Scopus Campus, Jerusalem, Israel,
[5]Kentucky Children's Hospital, University of Kentucky College of Medicine, Lexington, Kentucky, US,

[*] Correspondence: Ronald Chow BMSc(C), Infinitas Research GroupLondon, ON, Canada. Email: rchow48@uwo.ca.

[6]Center for Healthy Development, School of Public Health, Georgia State University, Atlanta, US

Parkinson's disease, first described by the English surgeon James Parkinson (1755-1824) in 1817 as "shaking palsy", is a neuro-degenerative disorder that manifests symptoms such as resting tremor, muscular rigidity, bradykinesia and postural instability. These motor disorders have been extensively researched resulting in improved diagnostic accuracy and development of robust rating scales and treatment strategies for symptoms. The treatment options for Parkinson's disease are similar to those for Alzheimer's disease, meaning that at this moment in time there does not exist a definitive cure that can reverse the progression of the disease. Young adults seems to be well aware of Alzheimer's disease, but are they aware of Parkinson's disease? Both of these diseases will become increasingly more prevalent in our aging world and young adults need to be prepared to care for family members who are struck by one, or both, diseases. In this book we document the assessment of the knowledge of young adults with respect to Parkinson's disease, across the globe.

INTRODUCTION

Parkinson's disease, first described by the English surgeon James Parkinson (1755-1824) in 1817 as "shaking palsy", is a neuro-degenerative disorder that manifests symptoms such as resting tremor, muscular rigidity, bradykinesia and postural instability (1-2). These motor disorders have been extensively researched resulting in improved diagnostic accuracy and development of robust rating scales and treatment strategies for symptoms (3-4).

In addition to motor problems, several non-motor features have also been noted - depression, psychosis, falls and sleep disturbances - that affect quality of life measures, institutionalization rates and health economics (5-12). This severity of symptoms is positively correlated with age and disease severity, and also precursors to olfactory problems and constipation (13).

With the average age and life expectancy of the population increasing, the non-motor symptoms of Parkinson's disease are becoming increasingly severe (13, 14). Coupled with the horrendous motor symptoms and also the lack of cure for the disease, the best form of treatment in addition to current pharmacological approaches to symptom treatment is to help improve quality of life of patients by understanding their sufferings.

The treatment options for Parkinson's disease are similar to those for Alzheimer's disease, meaning that at this moment in time there does not exist a definitive cure that can reverse the progression of the disease. Calls for research into awareness of Alzheimer's disease among young adults (15) has resulted in the documentation that young adults seem to be adequately aware of that disease (16).

Young adults have been shown to be well aware of Alzheimer's disease, but are they aware of Parkinson's disease? Both of these diseases will become increasingly more prevalent in our aging world, and young adults need to be prepared to care for family members who are struck by one, or both, diseases. The studies contained herein document the assessment of the knowledge of young adults with respect to Parkinson's disease, across the globe.

ACKNOWLEDGMENTS

We would like to thank Jaclyn Viehweger, Tharani Anpalagan, Victoria Trasente and Anna Rzepka for their support.

REFERENCES

[1] Parkinson J. An essay on the shaking palsy. London: Whitingham Rowland, 1817.

[2] Polymeropoulos MH, Lavedan C, Leroy E, Ide SE, Dehejia A, Dutra A, et al. Mutation in the α-Synuclein gene identified in families with Parkinson's disease. Science 1997;276(5321):2045-7.

[3] Hughes AJ, Daniel SE, Kilford L, Lees AJ. Accuracy of clinical diagnosis of idiopathic Parkinson's disease: a clinico-pathological study of 100 cases. J Neurol Neurosurg Psychiatry 1992;55:181-4.

[4] Fahn S, Elton RL, UPDRS Development Committee. Unified Parkinson's disease rating scale. In: Fahn S, Marsden CD, Calne D, Goldstein M, eds. Recent developments in Parkinson's disease. Florham Park, NJ: MacMillan Healthcare Information, 1987:153-63.

[5] Global Parkinson's Disease Survey Steering Committee. Factors impacting on quality of life in Parkinson's disease: results from an international survey. Mov Disord 2002;17:60-7.

[6] Chaudhuri KR, Schapira AHV, Martinez-Martin P. The holistic management of Parkinson's using a novel non-motor symptom scale and questionnaire. Adv Clin Neurosci Rehab 2004;4:20-4.

[7] Aarsland D, Larsen JP, Tandberg E, Laake K. Predictors of nursing home placement in Parkinson's disease: a population-based, prospective study. J Am Geriatr Soc 2000;48:938-42.

[8] Witjas T, Kaphan E, Azulay JP, Blin O, Ceccaldi M, Pouget J, et al. Nonmotor fluctuations in Parkinson's disease: frequent and disabling. Neurology 2002;59: 408-13.

[9] Schrag A, Jahanshahi N, Quinn N. What contributes to quality of life in patients with Parkinson's disease? J Neurol Neurosurg Psychiatry 2000;69:308-12.

[10] Findley L, Aujla M, Bain PG, Baker M, Beech C, Bowman C, et al. Direct economic impact of Parkinson's disease: a research survey in the United Kingdom. Mov Disord 2003;18:1139-45.

[11] Hagell P, Nordling S, Reimer J, Grabowski M, Persson U. Resource use and costs in a Swedish cohort of patients with Parkinson's disease. Mov Disord 2002;17:1213-20.

[12] Pressley JC, Louis ED, Tang MX, Cote L, Cohen PD, Glied S, et al. The impact of comorbid disease and injuries on resource use and expenditures in parkinsonism. Neurology 2003;60:87-93.

[13] Chaudhurri KR, Yates L, Martinex-Martin P. The non-motor symptom complex of Parkinson's disease: time for a comprehensive assessment. Curr Neurol Neurosci Rep 2005;5:275-83.

[14] Hely MA, Morris JGL, Reid WGL, Trafficante R. Sydney multicenter study of Parkinson's disease: Non-L-dopa-responsive problems dominate at 15 years. Mov Disord 2005;20:190-9.

[15] Chow R, Hollenberg D, Borean M, Merrick J, eds. Alzheimer's disease: Awareness among young adults. New York: Nova Science, 2017.

In: Parkinson's Disease
Editors: Ronald Chow, et al.
ISBN: 978-1-53612-745-4

Chapter 2

AWARENESS OF PARKINSON'S DISEASE: ABOUT THE SURVEY INSTRUMENT

Ronald Chow*, BMSc(C), Michael Borean, BMSc(C) and Drew Hollenberg, BMSc(C)
Infinitas Research Group, London, Ontario, Canada

The aim of our survey was to assess the perceived and actual awareness level of young adults. The survey was three pages and circulated via media outlets (i.e., email, social media). The first page was a consent form detailing why the study was done, the benefits/costs and other important information regarding the consent process. The second page collected demographic information of respondents. The questionnaire was marketed as voluntary and targeted towards young adults. The third page assessed the perceived and actual knowledge of participants. The first question assessed participant's perceived knowledge, and was an agree-neutral-disagree response to the statement that the participant was knowledgeable about Parkinson's disease. The subsequent eight

* Correspondence: Ronald Chow BMSc(C), Infinitas Research Group, Unit 1711-1235 Richmond St, London, ON N6A 0C1, Canada. Email: rchow48@uwo.ca.

questions were True-False questions to note the knowledge of participants.

Introduction

Parkinson's disease is projected to become increasingly more prevalent with the aging population (1, 2). Similar to the situation with Alzheimer's disease, there is no cure to reverse the disease, but only treatments for symptoms; hence, one of the best ways to improve quality of life in addition to pharmacological approaches is to increase the knowledge and awareness of family members and caregivers (3). The aim of our survey was to assess the perceived and actual awareness level of young adults.

Our survey

The survey was three pages (see figures 1-3) and circulated via media outlets (i.e., email, social media). The questionnaire was marketed as voluntary and targeted towards young adults, using the following text:

> Impaired movement, constant pain, never-ending tremor ...
>
> One million people are diagnosed with Parkinson's disease, costing an estimate of upwards of 25 billion per year to treat in the United States alone. These are very alarming numbers for a disease not many know much about. Infinitas Research Group has decided to assess the awareness of this disease across the globe.
>
> Please help us out and make this world a better place, by taking a few minutes to quickly fill out this survey: https://docs.google.com/forms/d/e/1FAIpQLSfO0cNPpZm-vJjSn8Qj5aFoBDOY6CZMfof7XFCbpDodZblzVA/viewform

The first page was a consent form detailing why the study was done, the benefits/costs and other important information regarding the consent process (see Figure 1). In order to progress from the first page to the second page, there was a question to document whether potential participants consent or do not consent to the study, of which participants must consent. If a person does not consent to the study, they finish the survey after page 1.

The second page collected demographic information of respondents. The questions asked participants to identify their primary place of location (i.e., where they live for the majority of the year), the age group they belong to, their sex, and whether they have family member(s) afflicted by Parkinson's disease. The last question on the page was applicable only to participants who had a family member afflicted, and asked them how many times a year they visit that family member (see Figure 2).

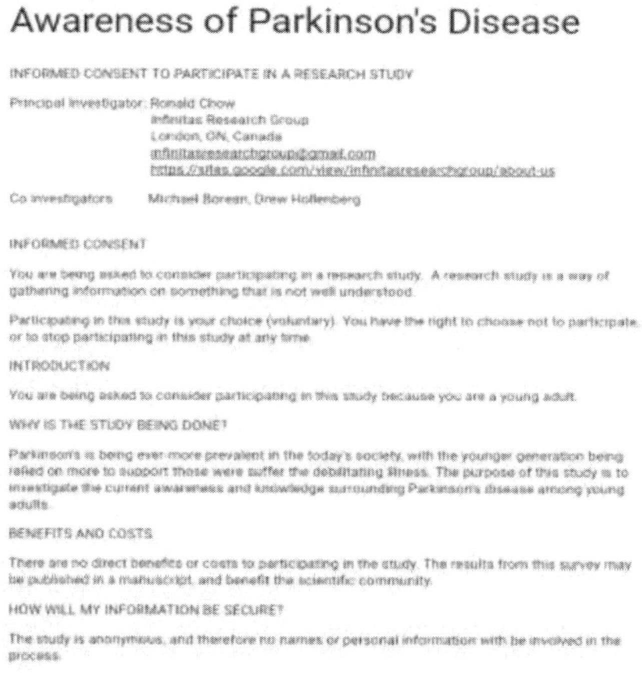

Awareness of Parkinson's Disease

INFORMED CONSENT TO PARTICIPATE IN A RESEARCH STUDY

Principal Investigator: Ronald Chow
Infinitas Research Group
London, ON, Canada
infinitasresearchgroup@gmail.com
https://sites.google.com/view/infinitasresearchgroup/about-us

Co investigators Michael Borean, Drew Hollenberg

INFORMED CONSENT

You are being asked to consider participating in a research study. A research study is a way of gathering information on something that is not well understood.

Participating in this study is your choice (voluntary). You have the right to choose not to participate or to stop participating in this study at any time.

INTRODUCTION

You are being asked to consider participating in this study because you are a young adult.

WHY IS THE STUDY BEING DONE?

Parkinson's is being ever-more prevalent in the today's society, with the younger generation being relied on more to support those were suffer the debilitating illness. The purpose of this study is to investigate the current awareness and knowledge surrounding Parkinson's disease among young adults.

BENEFITS AND COSTS

There are no direct benefits or costs to participating in the study. The results from this survey may be published in a manuscript, and benefit the scientific community.

HOW WILL MY INFORMATION BE SECURE?

The study is anonymous, and therefore no names or personal information with be involved in the process.

Figure 1. Survey (page 1).

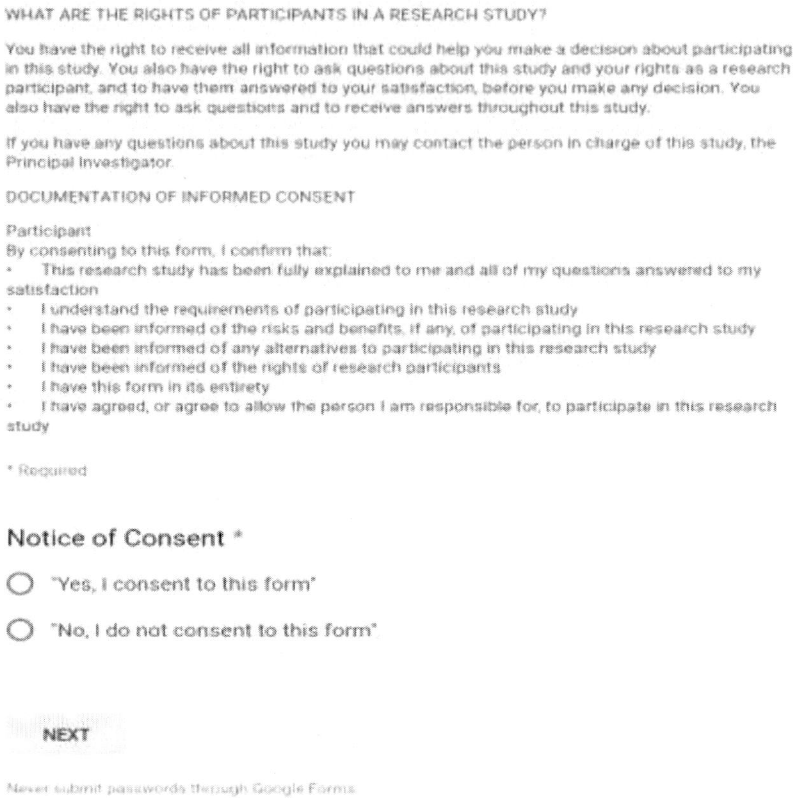

WHAT ARE THE RIGHTS OF PARTICIPANTS IN A RESEARCH STUDY?

You have the right to receive all information that could help you make a decision about participating in this study. You also have the right to ask questions about this study and your rights as a research participant, and to have them answered to your satisfaction, before you make any decision. You also have the right to ask questions and to receive answers throughout this study.

If you have any questions about this study you may contact the person in charge of this study, the Principal Investigator.

DOCUMENTATION OF INFORMED CONSENT

Participant
By consenting to this form, I confirm that:
- This research study has been fully explained to me and all of my questions answered to my satisfaction
- I understand the requirements of participating in this research study
- I have been informed of the risks and benefits, if any, of participating in this research study
- I have been informed of any alternatives to participating in this research study
- I have been informed of the rights of research participants
- I have this form in its entirety
- I have agreed, or agree to allow the person I am responsible for, to participate in this research study

* Required

Notice of Consent *

○ "Yes, I consent to this form"

○ "No, I do not consent to this form"

NEXT

Never submit passwords through Google Forms.

Figure 1. Survey (page 1).

The third page assessed the perceived and actual knowledge of participants. The first question assessed participant's perceived knowledge, and was a Agree-Neutral-Disagree response to the statement that the participant was knowledgeable about Parkinson's disease. The subsequent eight questions were True-False questions to note the knowledge of participants, with the answer being either True or False (see Figure 3). The answers to the questions are as follows:

1. "The cause of Parkinson's disease is unknown" - TRUE
2. "There is no cure to the disease, only treatments of symptoms" - TRUE

3. "There is no specific test to diagnose Parkinson's disease" - TRUE
4. "Stress can worsen the condition" - TRUE
5. "Exercise may slow the progression of Parkinson's disease" - TRUE
6. "Parkinson's only affects old people" - FALSE
7. "Men and women are equally as likely to be affected by Parkinson's" - FALSE
8. "There is no correlation between Parkinson's and depression" - FALSE

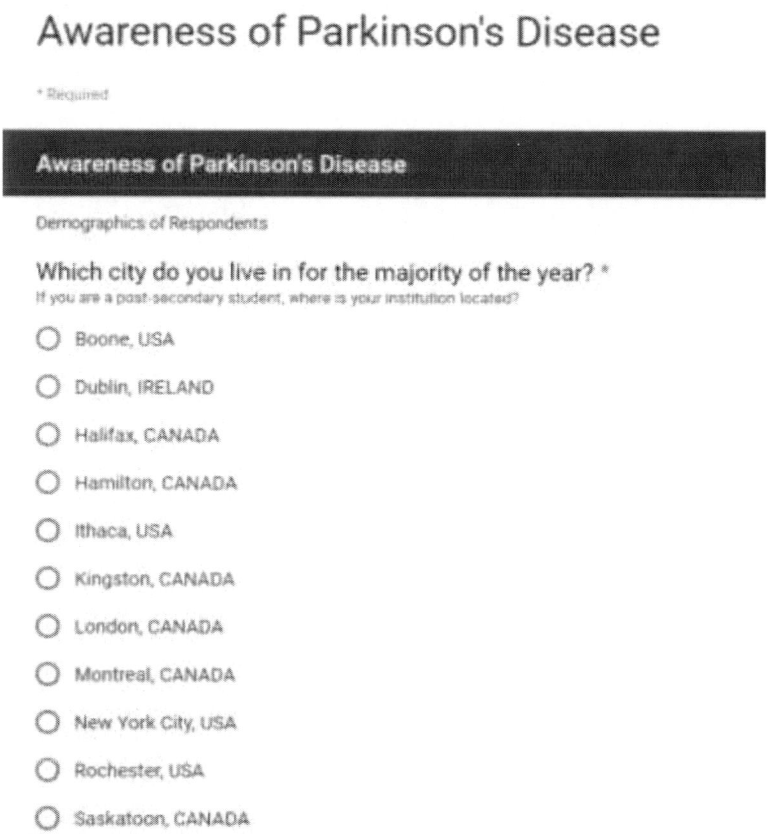

Awareness of Parkinson's Disease

* Required

Awareness of Parkinson's Disease

Demographics of Respondents

Which city do you live in for the majority of the year? *

If you are a post-secondary student, where is your institution located?

- Boone, USA
- Dublin, IRELAND
- Halifax, CANADA
- Hamilton, CANADA
- Ithaca, USA
- Kingston, CANADA
- London, CANADA
- Montreal, CANADA
- New York City, USA
- Rochester, USA
- Saskatoon, CANADA

Figure 2. Survey (page 2).

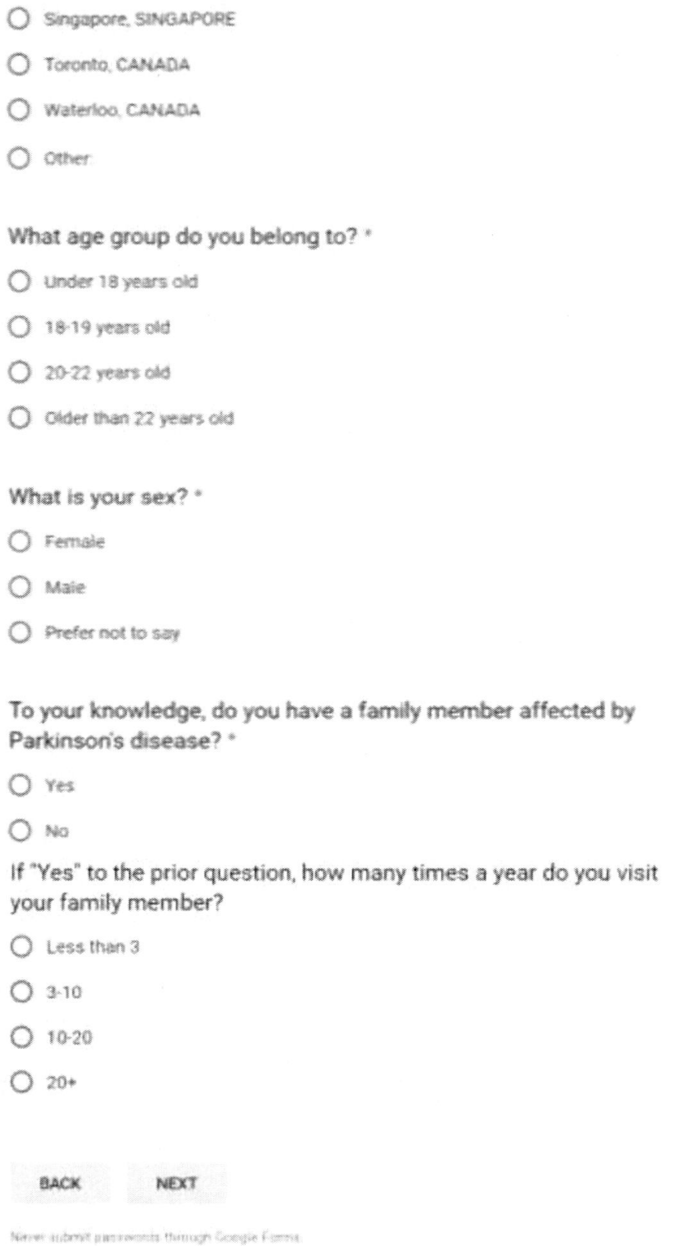

- Singapore, SINGAPORE
- Toronto, CANADA
- Waterloo, CANADA
- Other:

What age group do you belong to? *

- Under 18 years old
- 18-19 years old
- 20-22 years old
- Older than 22 years old

What is your sex? *

- Female
- Male
- Prefer not to say

To your knowledge, do you have a family member affected by Parkinson's disease? *

- Yes
- No

If "Yes" to the prior question, how many times a year do you visit your family member?

- Less than 3
- 3-10
- 10-20
- 20+

BACK NEXT

Never submit passwords through Google Forms.

Figure 2. Survey (page 2).

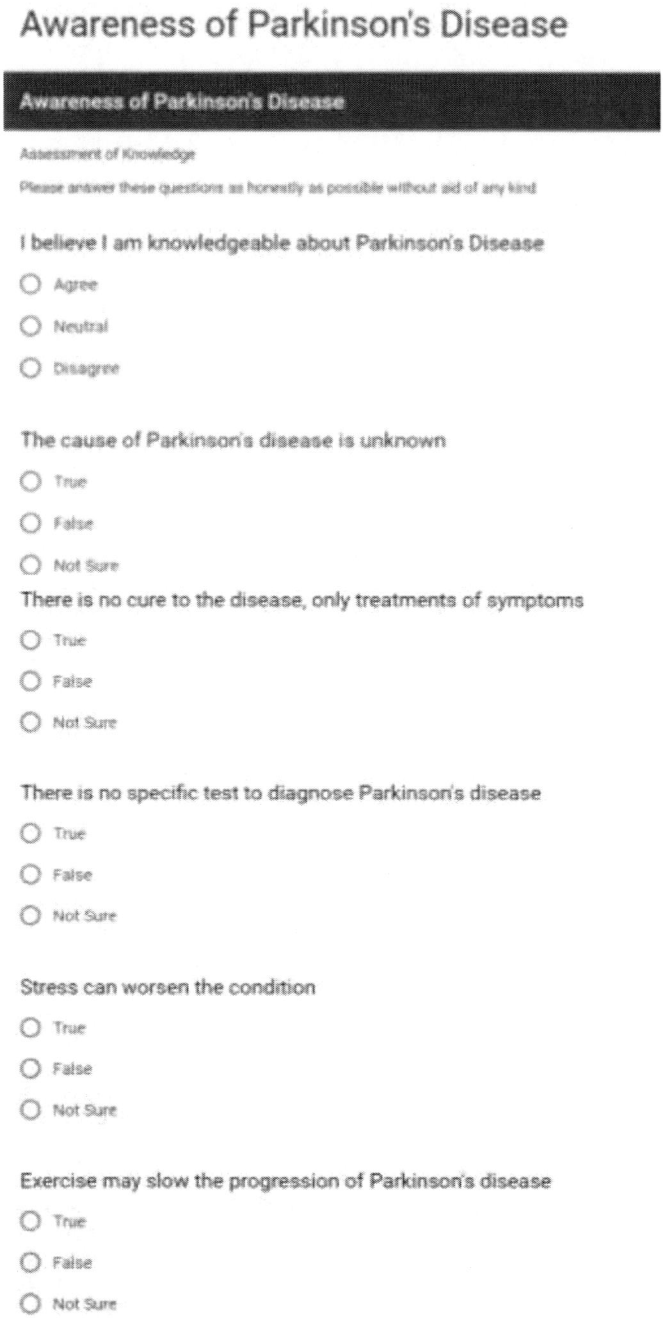

Awareness of Parkinson's Disease

Awareness of Parkinson's Disease

Assessment of Knowledge

Please answer these questions as honestly as possible without aid of any kind

I believe I am knowledgeable about Parkinson's Disease

- Agree
- Neutral
- Disagree

The cause of Parkinson's disease is unknown

- True
- False
- Not Sure

There is no cure to the disease, only treatments of symptoms

- True
- False
- Not Sure

There is no specific test to diagnose Parkinson's disease

- True
- False
- Not Sure

Stress can worsen the condition

- True
- False
- Not Sure

Exercise may slow the progression of Parkinson's disease

- True
- False
- Not Sure

Figure 3. Survey (page 3).

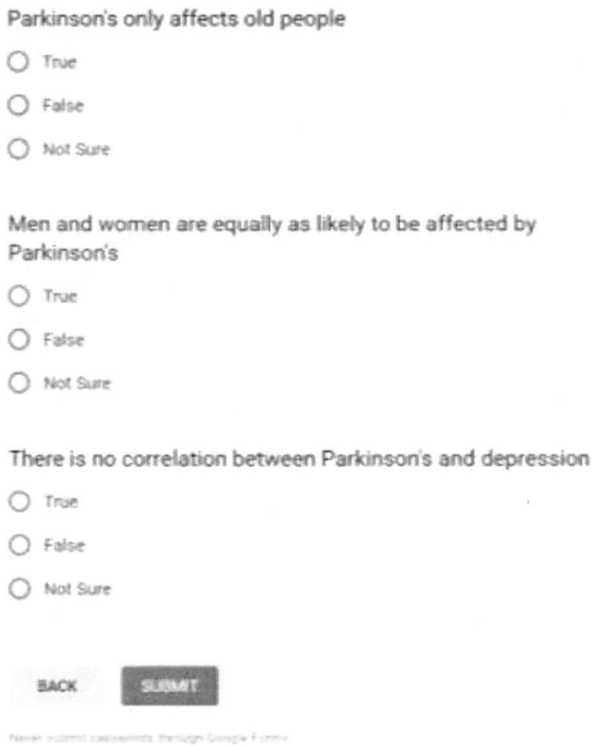
Parkinson's only affects old people

- True
- False
- Not Sure

Men and women are equally as likely to be affected by Parkinson's

- True
- False
- Not Sure

There is no correlation between Parkinson's and depression

- True
- False
- Not Sure

BACK SUBMIT

Figure 3. Survey (page 3).

Statistical analysis

Descriptive statistics were used to portray the participant demographics. For each participant, the number of correct answers was noted. The number of people who answered a question correctly was also recorded.

Fisher exact tests were used to compared the percentage of subgroups (age, gender, familial ties) who answered correctly/ incorrectly, and ANOVA procedures (using pooled means) were used to compare the average scores between the subgroups. P-values less than 0.05 were considered statistically significant. All statistical analyses were conducted using the Statistical Analysis Software (SAS Version 9.4 for Windows).

ACKNOWLEDGMENTS

We would like to thank Jaclyn Viehweger, Tharani Anpalagan, Victoria Trasente and Anna Rzepka in their support/help in designing the survey.

REFERENCES

[1] Chaudhurri KR, Yates L, Martinex-Martin P. The non-motor symptom complex of Parkinson's disease: time for a comprehensive assessment. Curr Neurol Neurosci Rep 2005;5:275-83.

[2] Hely MA, Morris JGL, Reid WGL, Trafficante R. Sydney multicenter study of Parkinson's disease: non-L-dopa-responsive problems dominate at 15 years. Mov Disord 2005;20:190-9.

[3] Chow R, Borean M, Hollenberg D, Merrick J. How aware/knowledgeable are young adults about Parkinson's disease? J Pain Manage 2019; in press.

SECTION ONE: CANADA

In: Parkinson's Disease
Editors: Ronald Chow, et al.
ISBN: 978-1-53612-745-4

Chapter 3

AWARENESS OF PARKINSON'S DISEASE AMONG YOUNG ADULTS IN LONDON, CANADA

Ronald Chow[1,*], BMSc(C), Jaclyn Viehweger[1], BMSc(C), Rachna Jog[2], HBA(C), Victoria Trasente[1], BA(C), Michael Borean[1], BMSc(C), Drew Hollenberg[1], BMSc(C), Michael Lam[1], BMSc(C), Tharani Anpalagan[1], BMSc(C) and Anna Rzepka[1], BMSc(C)

[1]Infinitas Research Group, London, Ontario, Canada
[2]Students Fight Parkinson's Western, London, Ontario, Canada

Parkinson's disease is a neurodegenerative disorder that has motor and non-motor symptoms. The aim of this study was to investigate the awareness, both perceived and actual, of young adults in London,

* Correspondence: Ronald Chow BMSc(C), Infinitas Research Group, London, Ontario, Canada. Email: rchow48@uwo.ca.

Ontario, Canada. A survey was circulated to young adults in London, Ontario, Canada via social media outlets. They were promoted as voluntary, and had no benefits/costs to participants. The first page had a consent form, second page collected information about participant demographics, and the third page contained nine questions to assess the participants' knowledge of Parkinson's disease. Fisher exact tests and ANOVA procedures were used to determine whether there was a difference in response between subgroups - age, gender and familial ties. 41% of participants believed that they were knowledgeable about the disease and 27% had family members, to their knowledge, affected by the disease. The actual awareness rate of 54% exceeds the other two statistics, reassuring us that young adults seem to be adequately aware. However, there still exists a large proportion of young adults who are not aware - education programs can be established to change this situation.

INTRODUCTION

Parkinson's disease is a neurodegenerative disorder that has motor and non-motor symptoms (1). Motor symptoms include resting tremor, muscular rigidity, bradykinesia and postural instability; non-motor symptoms include depression, psychosis, falls and sleep disturbances (2-10).

Parkinson's disease is becoming increasingly severe and more prevalent in our population. However, there is yet to exist a cure for Parkinson's disease. Given the projected increase in occurrence and the lack of cure, one of the best approaches to increase care and quality of life is to simply increase knowledge and awareness of caregivers so they can provide better holistic care (11). The aim of this study was to investigate the awareness, both perceived and actual, of young adults in London, Ontario, Canada.

Our study

A survey was circulated to young adults in London, Ontario, Canada via social media outlets. They were promoted as voluntary, and had no benefits/costs to participants. The first page had a consent form, second page collected information about participant demographics, and the third page contained nine questions to check the participants' knowledge of Parkinson's disease (12).

Descriptive statistics were used to disclose participant demographics. The number of correct answers were noted. Fisher exact tests and ANOVA procedures were used to determine whether there was a difference in response between subgroups - age, gender and familial ties. All analyses were conducted using the Statistical Analysis Software (SAS Version 9.4 for Windows) (12).

Findings

The majority (66%) of the 41 participants were between 18 and 19 years old; 24% were between 20 and 22 years old, 5% were under 18 years old, and 5% were over 22 years old. Four-fifths remarked that they are female, and the remainder noted they are male. 11 (27%), to their knowledge, have a family member affected by Parkinson's disease. Of these 11 participants, 6 (55%) visited their family member more than 20 times a year, 18% between 10 to 12 times a year, 18% between 3 and 10 times a year, and 9% less than 3 times a year (see Table 1).

Table 1. Demographics

Demographic	n = 41
Age Group	
Under 18 years old	2 (5%)
18-19 years old	27 (66%)
20-22 years old	10 (24%)
Over 22 years old	2 (5%)
Sex	
Male	8 (20%)
Female	33 (80%)
Prefer not to say	0 (0%)
Family member affected by Parkinson's disease	
Yes	11 (27%)
No	30 (73%)
Number of visits to Parkinson's family member a year (n = 11)	
Less than 3	1 (9%)
3-10	2 (18%)
10-20	2 (18%)
20+	6 (55%)

41% of participants believe that they are knowledgeable about Parkinson's disease, 22% reserved judgement, and 37% believed they are not knowledgeable. 32% correctly answered that Parkinson's disease has an unknown cause, 90% properly remarked that there is no cure to the disease, and 29% responded that there is indeed no specific test to diagnose Parkinson's. 76% answered that stress can worsen the condition, 59% noted that exercise slows the progression of Parkinson's, 93% note that it does not only affect old people, 37% believe that it does not equally affect men and women, and 51% correctly answered that there is no correlation between Parkinson's and depression. Overall, 20% were knowledgeable, 34% had satisfactory knowledge, and 46% were not knowledgeable about Parkinson's disease. The average score was 4.66 out of 8 (see Table 2).

Table 2. Perceived and actual knowledge

Question Item	n = 41
"I believe I am knowledgeable about Parkinson's disease"	
Agree	17 (41%)
Disagree	9 (22%)
Neutral	15 (37%)
"The cause of Parkinson's disease is unknown"	
True	13 (32%)
False	13 (32%)
Not Sure	15 (37%)
"There is no cure to the disease, only treatments of symptoms"	
True	37 (90%)
False	0 (0%)
Not Sure	4 (10%)
"There is no specific test to diagnose Parkinson's disease"	
True	12 (29%)
False	14 (34%)
Not Sure	15 (37%)
"Stress can worsen the condition"	
True	31 (76%)
False	1 (2%)
Not Sure	9 (22%)
"Exercise may slow the progression of Parkinson's disease"	
True	24 (59%)
False	5 (12%)
Not Sure	12 (29%)
"Parkinson's only affects old people"	
True	0 (0%)
False	38 (93%)
Not Sure	3 (7%)
"Men and women are equally as likely to be affected by Parkinson's"	
True	
False	9 (22%)
Not Sure	15 (37%)
	17 (42%)
"There is no correlation between Parkinson's and depression"	
True	2 (5%)
False	21 (51%)
Not Sure	18 (44%)
Knowledge Score	
Not Knowledgeable (0-4)	19 (46%)
Satisfactory (5-6)	14 (34%)
Knowledgeable (7-8)	8 (20%)
Mean ± SD	4.66 ± 1.80

There were no significant differences in responses by the younger (under 20 years old) and older (over 20 years old) cohorts. 38% of the younger and 50% of the older remarked that they were knowledgeable about the disease (p = 0.8255). 34% and 25%, respectively, answered that there is no cause for Parkinson's disease (p = 0.3241); 90% and 92% noted that there is no cure to the disease (p = 0.9999), 28% and 33% answered that there is no specific diagnostic test (p = 0.6860), and 72% and 83% recorded that stress worsens the condition (p = 0.1854). 59% and 58% remarked that exercise may slow the progression (p = 0.7891), 90% and 100% answered that Parkinson's does not only affect old people (p = 0.5430), 17% and 33% incorrectly noted that men and women are equally affected (p = 0.3074), and 55% and 42% correctly noted that there is a correlation between Parkinson's and depression (p = 0.6286). Overall, 48% and 42% were not knowledgeable (p = 0.3638), and the mean scores were 4.60 and 4.75 out of 8 (p = 0.8114) (see Table 3).

Table 3. Perceived and actual knowledge - by subgroups

Question Item	**Under 20 n = 29**	**Over 20 n = 12**	**p-value**
"I believe I am knowledgeable about Parkinson's disease"			0.8255
Agree	11 (38%)	6 (50%)	
Disagree	7 (24%)	2 (17%)	
Neutral	11 (38%)	4 (33%)	
"The cause of Parkinson's disease is unknown"			0.3241
True	10 (34%)	3 (25%)	
False	7 (24%)	6 (50%)	
Not Sure	12 (41%)	3 (25%)	
"There is no cure to the disease, only treatments of			0.9999
symptoms"	26 (90%)	11 (92%)	
True	0 (0%)	0 (0%)	
False	3 (10%)	1 (8%)	
Not Sure			

Question Item	Under 20 n = 29	Over 20 n = 12	p-value
"There is no specific test to diagnose Parkinson's disease"			0.6860
True	8 (28%)	4 (33%)	
False	9 (31%)	5 (42%)	
Not Sure	12 (41%)	3 (25%)	
"Stress can worsen the condition"			0.1854
True	21 (72%)	10 (83%)	
False	0 (0%)	1 (8%)	
Not Sure	8 (28%)	1 (8%)	
"Exercise may slow the progression of Parkinson's disease"			0.7891
True	17 (59%)	7 (58%)	
False	3 (10%)	2 (17%)	
Not Sure	9 (31%)	3 (25%)	
"Parkinson's only affects old people"			0.5430
True	0 (0%)	0 (0%)	
False	26 (90%)	12 (100%)	
Not Sure	3 (10%)	0 (0%)	
"Men and women are equally as likely to be affected by Parkinson's"			0.3074
True	5 (17%)	4 (33%)	
False	10 (34%)	5 (42%)	
Not Sure	14 (48%)	3 (25%)	
"There is no correlation between Parkinson's and depression"			0.6286
True	1 (3%)	1 (8%)	
False	16 (55%)	5 (42%)	
Not Sure	12 (41%)	6 (50%)	
Knowledge Score			
Not Knowledgeable (0-4)	14 (48%)	5 (42%)	0.3638
Satisfactory (5-6)	8 (28%)	6 (50%)	
Knowledgeable (7-8)	7 (24%)	1 (8%)	
Mean ± SD	4.60 ± 1.97	4.75 ± 1.36	0.8114
Question Item	**Males n = 8**	**Females n = 33**	
"I believe I am knowledgeable about Parkinson's disease"			0.2127
Agree	5 (63%)	12 (36%)	
Disagree	0 (0%)	9 (27%)	
Neutral	3 (37%)	12 (36%)	

Table 3. (Continued)

Question Item	Males n = 8	Females n = 33	
"The cause of Parkinson's disease is unknown"			0.5494
True	4 (50%)	9 (27%)	
False	2 (25%)	11 (33%)	
Not Sure	2 (25%)	13 (39%)	
"There is no cure to the disease, only treatments of symptoms"			0.5690
True	8 (100%)	29 (88%)	
False	0 (0%)	0 (0%)	
Not Sure	0 (0%)	4 (12%)	
"There is no specific test to diagnose Parkinson's disease"			0.9999
True	2 (25%)	10 (30%)	
False	3 (37%)	11 (33%)	
Not Sure	3 (37%)	12 (36%)	
"Stress can worsen the condition"			0.9999
True	6 (75%)	25 (76%)	
False	0 (0%)	1 (3%)	
Not Sure	2 (25%)	7 (21%)	
"Exercise may slow the progression of Parkinson's disease"			0.1312
True	7 (88%)	17 (52%)	
False	1 (13%)	4 (12%)	
Not Sure	0 (0%)	12 (36%)	
"Parkinson's only affects old people"			0.4882
True	0 (0%)	0 (0%)	
False	7 (88%)	31 (94%)	
Not Sure	1 (13%)	2 (6%)	
"Men and women are equally as likely to be affected by Parkinson's"			0.7814
True	2 (25%)	7 (21%)	
False	2 (25%)	13 (39%)	
Not Sure	4 (50%)	13 (39%)	
"There is no correlation between Parkinson's and depression"			0.3262
True	1 (13%)	1 (3%)	
False	3 (38%)	18 (55%)	
Not Sure	4 (50%)	14 (43%)	

Question Item	Males n = 8	Females n = 33	
Knowledge Score Not Knowledgeable (0-4) Satisfactory (5-6) Knowledgeable (7-8) Mean ± SD	 5 (63%) 1 (13%) 2 (25%) 4.89 ± 1.89	 14 (43%) 13 (39%) 6 (18%) 4.61 ± 1.80	 0.4035 0.6978
Question Item	**Affected n = 11**	**Unaffected n = 30**	
"I believe I am knowledgeable about Parkinson's disease" Agree Disagree Neutral	7 (64%) 3 (27%) 1 (9%)	10 (33%) 8 (27%) 12 (40%)	0.1146
"The cause of Parkinson's disease is unknown" True False Not Sure	4 (36%) 4 (36%) 3 (27%)	9 (30%) 9 (30%) 12 (40%)	0.7456
"There is no cure to the disease, only treatments of symptoms" True False Not Sure	11 (100%) 0 (0%) 0 (0%)	26 (87%) 0 (0%) 4 (13%)	0.5590
"There is no specific test to diagnose Parkinson's disease" True False Not Sure	4 (36%) 1 (9%) 6 (55%)	8 (27%) 13 (43%) 9 (30%)	0.1083
"Stress can worsen the condition" True False Not Sure	9 (82%) 0 (0%) 2 (18%)	22 (73%) 1 (3%) 7 (23%)	0.9999
"Exercise may slow the progression of Parkinson's disease" True False Not Sure	7 (64%) 1 (9%) 3 (27%)	17 (57%) 4 (13%) 9 (30%)	0.9999
"Parkinson's only affects old people" True False Not Sure	0 (0%) 11 (100%) 0 (0%)	0 (0%) 27 (90%) 3 (10%)	0.5511

Table 3. (Continued)

Question Item	**Affected n = 11**	**Unaffected n = 30**	
"Men and women are equally as likely to be affected by Parkinson's"			0.6611
True	2 (18%)	7 (23%)	
False	3 (27%)	12 (40%)	
Not Sure	6 (55%)	11 (37%)	
"There is no correlation between Parkinson's and depression"			0.7333
True	0 (0%)	2 (7%)	
False	7 (64%)	14 (47%)	
Not Sure	4 (36%)	14 (47%)	
Knowledge Score			
Not Knowledgeable (0-4)	5 (45%)	14 (47%)	0.8093
Satisfactory (5-6)	3 (27%)	11 (37%)	
Knowledgeable (7-8)	3 (27%)	5 (17%)	
Mean ± SD	5.09 ± 1.58	4.50 ± 1.87	0.3582
Question Item	**Less than 10 visits n = 3**	**More than 10 visits n = 8**	
"I believe I am knowledgeable about Parkinson's disease"			0.6182
Agree	3 (100%)	4 (50%)	
Disagree	0 (0%)	1 (13%)	
Neutral	0 (0%)	3 (38%)	
"The cause of Parkinson's disease is unknown"			0.4182
True	0 (0%)	4 (50%)	
False	2 (67%)	2 (25%)	
Not Sure	1 (33%)	2 (25%)	
"There is no cure to the disease, only treatments of symptoms"	3 (100%)	8 (100%)	0.9999
True	0 (0%)	0 (0%)	
False	0 (0%)	0 (0%)	
Not Sure			
"There is no specific test to diagnose Parkinson's disease"			0.6364
True	2 (67%)	2 (25%)	
False	0 (0%)	1 (13%)	
Not Sure	1 (33%)	5 (63%)	

Question Item	Affected n = 11	Unaffected n = 30	
"Stress can worsen the condition"			0.9999
True	3 (100%)	6 (75%)	
False	0 (0%)	0 (0%)	
Not Sure	0 (0%)	2 (25%)	
"Exercise may slow the progression of Parkinson's			0.9999
disease"	2 (67%)	5 (63%)	
True	0 (0%)	1 (13%)	
False	1 (33%)	2 (25%)	
Not Sure			
"Parkinson's only affects old people"			0.9999
True	0 (0%)	0 (0%)	
False	3 (100%)	8 (100%)	
Not Sure	0 (0%)	0 (0%)	
"Men and women are equally as likely to be affected by Parkinson's"			0.2061
True	0 (0%)	2 (25%)	
False	2 (67%)	1 (13%)	
Not Sure	1 (33%)	5 (63%)	
"There is no correlation between Parkinson's and			0.9999
depression"	0 (0%)	0 (0%)	
True	2 (67%)	5 (63%)	
False	1 (33%)	3 (38%)	
Not Sure			
Knowledge Score			
Not Knowledgeable (0-4)	1 (33%)	4 (50%)	0.9999
Satisfactory (5-6)	1 (33%)	2 (25%)	
Knowledgeable (7-8)	1 (33%)	2 (25%)	
Mean ± SD	5.67 ± 1.53	4.88 ±1.64	0.4886

There were also no differences in responses between the sexes. 63% of males and 36% of females believe they are knowledgeable ($p = 0.2127$). 50% and 27% of the same groups, respectively, noted that the cause of Parkinson's disease is unknown ($p = 0.5494$), 100% and 88% remarked that there is no cure to the disease ($p = 0.5690$), 25% and 30% noted that there is no diagnostic test for Parkinson's ($p = 0.9999$), 75% and 76% reported that stress can worsen the condition ($p = 0.9999$),

88% and 52% noted that exercise can slow the progression (p = 0.1312), 88% and 94% answered that it does not only plague older individuals, 25% and 39% correctly noted that it does not affect men and women equally (p = 0.7814), and 38% and 55% reported that there is a correlation between Parkinson's and depression (p = 0.3262). With respect to the overall score, 63% and 43% were not knowledgeable (p = 0.4035), and the average scores were 4.89 and 4.61 (0.6978) (see Table 3).

Those who have and do not have a family member affected by Parkinson's disease had similar perceived and actual awareness. While 64% of those affected believed they were aware of the disease, 33% of those unaffected had a similar belief (p = 0.1146). 36% and 30% of the same cohorts noted that there is no known cause to the disease (p = 0.7456), 100% and 87% noted that there is no cure to the disease (p = 0.5590), 36% and 27% answered that there is no specific test (p = 0.1083), and 82% and 73% remarked that stress can worsen the condition (p = 0.9999). 64% and 57% accurately answered that exercise may slow the progression (p = 0.9999), while 100% and 90%, 27% and 40%, and 64% and 47% answered that Parkinson's does not only affect old people, the two sexes are not equally affected, and that there is a correlation between Parkinson's and depression, respectively. 45% and 47% of the two groups were not knowledgeable (p = 0.8093), and the average total scores were 5.09 and 4.50 (p = 0.3582) (see Table 3).

When comparing those who have family members affected by the disease by frequency of visiting the family member, there exists no difference in awareness. 100% and 50% of those who visit less than 10 times a year and more than 10 times a year, respectively, remarked that they were knowledgeable (p = 0.6182). 0% and 50% answered that the cause of Parkinson's disease is unknown (p = 0.4182), 100% and 100% noted that there is no cure to the disease (p = 0.9999), 67% and 25% remarked that there is no specific diagnostic test (p = 0.6364), 100% and 75% answered that stress can worsen the condition (p = 0.9999), and 67% and 63% reported that exercise may slow the progression of the disease (p = 0.9999). All of both groups, 0% and 25%, and 0% of both groups answered that Parkinson's does not only affect old people (p = 0.9999), that men and women are equally affected, and that there is no correlation between Parkinson's and depression (p = 0.9999). 33% and 25% were knowledgeable, and a same proportion had satisfactory knowledge (p = 0.9999); the average scores for the two groups were 5.67 and 4.88 out of 8 (p = 0.4886) (see Table 3).

DISCUSSION

This is the first study to our knowledge to survey the awareness, both perceived and actual, of young adults with respect to Parkinson's disease. Prior studies have been conducted among young adults but evaluating their awareness of Alzheimer's disease (13-15). Only 20% of participants were deemed knowledgeable of Parkinson's, which is remarkably lower than the awareness of young adults with respect to Alzheimer's. Programs should be established to increase the awareness and knowledge of Parkinson's, as it too is a very prevalent and burdensome disease in our communities.

The perceived awareness level (41% awareness) is lower than the actual awareness of 54% - 34% satisfactory knowledge and 20% knowledgeable. Coupled with the fact that only 11 of 41 respondents (27%) have family members affected by the disease, the awareness of young adults seems to be adequate in today's society. However, there still exists a large proportion of young adults who are not aware - education programs can be established to change this situation.

There also seems to be no inherent differences in awareness between males and females, between older and younger individuals, between those who have and do not have a family member affected, and between those who frequently and do not regularly visit their family member. The lack of noticeable difference, however, may be a result of the small sample size in the subgroup analyses - descriptive statistics suggest a difference but a very small sample size with low statistical power could not detect a statistical difference. Further studies with larger sample sizes should be conducted to determine whether there exists a difference between subgroups.

This study was not without limitations. As with any survey study, there exists the possibility of a sample/response bias. Additionally, the small sample size at times led to low statistical power, in particular to the subgroup analyses.

In conclusion, 41% of participants believed that they were knowledgeable about the disease and 27% had family members, to their knowledge, affected by the disease. The actual awareness rate of 54% exceeds the other two statistics, reassuring us that young adults seem to be adequately aware. However, there still exists a large proportion of young adults who are not aware - education programs can be established to change this situation.

ACKNOWLEDGMENTS

We would like to thank all respondents who participated in our study.

REFERENCES

[1] Parkinson J. An essay on the shaking palsy. London: Whitingham Rowland, 1817.

[2] Polymeropoulos MH, Lavedan C, Leroy E, Ide SE, Dehejia A, Dutra A, et al. Mutation in the α-synuclein gene identified in families with Parkinson's disease. Science 1997;276(5321):2045-7.

[3] Global Parkinson's Disease Survey Steering Committee. Factors impacting on quality of life in Parkinson's disease: results from an international survey. Mov Disord 2002;17:60-7.

[4] Chaudhuri KR, Schapira AHV, Martinez-Martin P. The holistic management of Parkinson's using a novel non-motor symptom scale and questionnaire. Adv Clin Neurosci Rehabil 2004;4:20-4.

[5] Aarsland D, Larsen JP, Tandberg E, Laake K. Predictors of nursing home placement in Parkinson's disease: a population-based, prospective study. J Am Geriatr Soc 2000;48:938-42.

[6] Witjas T, Kaphan E, Azulay JP, Blin O, Ceccaldi M, Pouget J, et al. Nonmotor fluctuations in Parkinson's disease: frequent and disabling. Neurology 2002;59:408-13.

[7] Schrag A, Jahanshahi N, Quinn N. What contributes to quality of life in patients with Parkinson's disease? J Neurol Neurosurg Psychiatry 2000;69:308-12.

[8] Findley L, Aujla M, Bain PG, Baker M, Beech C, Bowman C, et al. Direct economic impact of Parkinson's disease: a research survey in the United Kingdom. Mov Disord 2003;18:1139-45.

[9] Hagell P, Nordling S, Reimer J, Grabowski M, Persson U. Resource use and costs in a Swedish cohort of patients with Parkinson's disease. Mov Disord 2002;17:1213-20.

[10] Pressley JC, Louis ED, Tang MX, Cote L, Cohen PD, Glied S, et al. The impact of comorbid disease and injuries on resource use and expenditures in Parkinsonism. Neurology 2003;60:87-93.

[11] Chow R, Borean M, Hollenberg D, Merrick J. How aware/knowledgeable are young adults about Parkinson's disease? J Pain Manage 2019;12(1), in press.

[12] Chow R, Borean M, Hollenberg D. Awareness of Parkinson's disease: About the survey instrument. J Pain Manage 2019;12(1), in press.

[13] Chow R, Borean M, Hollenberg D, Merrick J. How knowledgeable are young adults about Alzheimer's disease? Int J Child Health Hum Dev 2018;11(4), in press.

[14] Chow R, Ferrara A, Borean M, Hollenberg D, Lam M, Anpalagan T, et al. Awareness of Alzheimer's disease among young adults in London, Canada. Int J Child Health Hum Dev 2018, in press.

[15] Chow R, Borean M, Hollenberg D, Midroni L, Midroni C, Kim Y, et al. Awareness of Alzheimer's disease among young adults in Kingston, Canada. Int J Child Health Hum Dev 2018, in press.

In: Parkinson's Disease
Editors: Ronald Chow, et al.
ISBN: 978-1-53612-745-4

Chapter 4

AWARENESS OF PARKINSON'S DISEASE AMONG YOUNG ADULTS IN TORONTO, CANADA

Stephanie Ho, Jaclyn Viehweger, BMSc(C), Victoria Trasente, BA(C), Cynthia Ho, BA(C), Wesley Ng, BSc(C), Matthew Wong, BA AS(C), Michael Borean, BMSc(C), Drew Hollenberg, BMSc(C), Tharani Anpalagan, BMSc(C), Anna Rzepka, BMSc(C) and Ronald Chow*, BMSc(C)
Infinitas Research Group, London, Ontario, Canada

Parkinson's disease is a debilitating illness that drastically affects quality of life, and unfortunately has no cure. The aim of this chapter was to hence determine the perceived/actual awareness of young adults in Toronto, Ontario, Canada. A survey was sent out via social media outlets to young adults in Toronto, Ontario, Canada. A total of 26 consenting

* Correspondence: Ronald Chow BMSc(C), Infinitas Research Group, London, Ontario, Canada. Email: rchow48@uwo.ca.

participants were included in our study. 35% of the young adults in Toronto, Canada, were aware of the disease. This number is higher than the 23% of young adults who have a family member affected by the disease and only 15% believe that they are knowledgeable, suggesting that young adults are adequately aware to take care of individuals with Parkinson's disease. The results also show that there exists variation in awareness by geographic region, and further studies should be conducted to investigate awareness in other regions.

INTRODUCTION

Parkinson's disease is a debilitating illness that drastically affects quality of life (QOL), and unfortunately has no cure (1-3). The motor and nonmotor symptoms such as tremors, muscular rigidity, bradykinesia, postural instability, depression, psychosis and sleep disturbances can noticeably decrease QOL in affected patients (4-10).

One of the best ways to help improve QOL of patients affected by Parkinson's, in addition to pharmacological therapies, is to increase awareness/knowledge of caregivers so that they can provide better holistic/patient-centred care (3). It is especially important for young adults to be aware, as these individuals will be those who will take care of the future population of our society where Parkinson's will be increasingly more prevalent.

An original survey study was conducted by Chow et al. to assess the perceived and actual awareness of young adults in London, Ontario, Canada. A survey was circulated to young adults in London and had eight questions designed to determine the knowledge of young adults about Parkinson's disease. The results of the survey revealed that 54% of young adults are aware of Parkinson's disease, which is lower than the awareness level of Alzheimer's disease that was published in prior studies. However, the 54% awareness rate is still in excess of the 41% of participants who believe they are knowledgeable and 27% who actually had a family member affected by the disease (11).

It is important to note that there may exist variation in awareness in different regions, as a result of the different prevalence and public perception of the disease in different regions. The aim of this study was to hence determine the perceived/actual awareness of young adults in Toronto, Ontario, Canada.

THE SURVEY

A survey was sent out via social media outlets to young adults in Toronto, Ontario, Canada. The survey was voluntary and the consent form on the first page acknowledged that there are no benefits/costs to participants. The second page collected demographic information and the third page was used to determine the actual and perceived awareness of Parkinson's disease (12).

Descriptive statistics were used to share participant demographics, and the number of correct/incorrect answers. Fisher exact tests were used to determine whether there was a difference in categorical questions between age groups (under and over 20 years old), gender groups (males and females), familial ties (affected and not affected by Parkinson's disease) and the frequency of visiting their family members (less than and over 10 visits a year). ANOVA procedures compared the average number of correct answers between the subgroups. All analyses were conducted using the Statistical Analysis Software (SAS Version 9.4 for Windows) (12).

FINDINGS

A total of 26 consenting participants were included in our study. 65% were 18-19 years old, 23% were between 20 and 22 years old, 8% were under 18 years old, and 4% were over 22 years old. The majority of participants identified as female (77%) and did not have a family member affected by Parkinson's disease (73%). Of the 7 participants who had family members affected by Parkinson's disease, 14% visited their family members more than 20 times a year, with the remaining participants split equally across less than 3, 3-10 and 10-20 visits a year (see Table 1).

Table 1. Demographics

Demographic	n = 26
Age Group	
Under 18 years old	2 (8%)
18-19 years old	17 (65%)
20-22 years old	6 (23%)
Over 22 years old	1 (4%)
Sex	
Male	6 (23%)
Female	20 (77%)
Prefer not to say	0 (0%)
Family member affected by Parkinson's disease	
Yes	7 (27%)
No	19 (73%)
Number of visits to Parkinson's family member a year (n = 7)	
Less than 3	2 (29%)
3-10	2 (29%)
10-20	2 (29%)
20+	1 (14%)

15% believed they were knowledgeable about Parkinson's disease; 35% claimed they were unknowledgeable and 50% reserved judgement. 31% correctly answered that the cause of Parkinson's disease is unknown, 88% acknowledged that there is no cure to the disease, 12% answered that there is no specific test to the disease, and 77% noted that stress can indeed worsen the condition. 62% accurately noted that exercise may slow the progression of Parkinson's disease, 96% answered that it does not only affect old people, 23% noted that men and women are not equally likely to be affected and 42% reported that there is a correlation between Parkinson's and depression. Overall, 12%

were deemed knowledgeable and 23% had satisfactory knowledge, and the average score was 4.31 out of 8 (see Table 2).

There was a trend that those over 20 years old believed they were more knowledgeable about the disease ($p = 0.0821$) - 29% reported they were knowledgeable compared to 11% for the other age cohort. In reality, there were no differences in awareness between the two groups. 37% and 14% of those under 20 and over 20 years old, respectively, noted that there is no cause to Parkinson's disease ($p = 0.5174$); 84% and 100% noted that there is no cure ($p = 0.9999$), 11% and 14% answered that there is no specific diagnostic test ($p = 0.9999$), 84% and 57% correctly identified that stress can worsen the condition ($p = 0.2929$), and 63% and 57% responded that exercise can slow the progression of the disease ($p = 0.9999$). 95% and 100% correctly identified that Parkinson's does not only affect old people ($p = 0.9999$), 26% and 14% incorrectly believed that men and women are equally affected by the disease ($p = 0.1240$) and 47% and 29% correctly believed that there is a correlation between Parkinson's and depression ($p = 0.6576$). 63% and 71% were not knowledgeable, overall ($p = 0.6576$), and the average scores for the younger and older cohorts were 4.53 and 3.71, respectively ($p = 0.2106$) (see Table 3).

With respect to males and females, there exists no difference in perceived and actual awareness level. 17% and 15% of males and females, respectively, believed that they were knowledgeable about Parkinson's disease ($p = 0.7073$). The same two cohorts noted, at 33% and 30% frequency, that the cause of Parkinson's is unknown ($p = 0.6025$); 100% and 85% reported that there is no cure to the disease ($p = 0.9999$), 67% and 50% answered that there is no specific test to diagnose Parkinson's disease ($p = 0.8292$), 50% and 85% noted that stress can worsen the condition ($p = 0.1119$), and 50% and 65% identified that exercise may slow the progression ($p = 0.3819$). 100% and 95% reported that it does not only affect old people ($p = 0.9999$), 17% and 25% noted that men and women are not equally affected ($p = 0.3395$), and 50% and 40% answered that there is a correlation between Parkinson's and depression (p = 0.6739). 67% and 65^ were not knowledgeable about the disease (p = 0.9999), and the average score for the two groups were 4.00 and 4.40, respectively (p = 0.5676) (see Table 3).

Table 2. Perceived and actual knowledge

Question Item	**n = 26**
"I believe I am knowledgeable about Parkinson's disease"	
Agree	4 (15%)
Disagree	9 (35%)
Neutral	13 (50%)
"The cause of Parkinson's disease is unknown"	
True	8 (31%)
False	5 (19%)
Not Sure	13 (50%)
"There is no cure to the disease, only treatments of symptoms"	
True	23 (88%)
False	1 (4%)
Not Sure	2 (8%)
"There is no specific test to diagnose Parkinson's disease"	
True	3 (12%)
False	14 (54%)
Not Sure	9 (35%)
"Stress can worsen the condition"	
True	20 (77%)
False	0 (0%)
Not Sure	6 (23%)
"Exercise may slow the progression of Parkinson's disease"	
True	16 (62%)
False	3 (12%)
Not Sure	7 (27%)
"Parkinson's only affects old people"	
True	1 (4%)
False	25 (96%)
Not Sure	0 (0%)
"Men and women are equally as likely to be affected by Parkinson's"	
True	6 (23%)
False	6 (23%)
Not Sure	14 (54%)

Question Item	n = 26
"There is no correlation between Parkinson's and depression"	
True	0 (0%)
False	11 (42%)
Not Sure	15 (58%)
Knowledge Score	
Not Knowledgeable (0-4)	17 (65%)
Satisfactory (5-6)	6 (23%)
Knowledgeable (7-8)	3 (12%)
Mean ± SD	4.31 ± 1.46

Table 3. Perceived and actual knowledge - by subgroups

Question Item	Under 20 n = 19	Over 20 n = 7	p-value
"I believe I am knowledgeable about Parkinson's disease"			0.0821
Agree	2 (11%)	2 (29%)	
Disagree	5 (26%)	4 (57%)	
Neutral	12 (63%)	1 (14%)	
"The cause of Parkinson's disease is unknown"			0.5174
True	7 (37%)	1 (14%)	
False	4 (21%)	1 (14%)	
Not Sure	8 (42%)	5 (71%)	
"There is no cure to the disease, only treatments of symptoms"			0.9999
True	16 (84%)	7 (100%)	
False	1 (5%)	0 (0%)	
Not Sure	2 (11%)	0 (0%)	
"There is no specific test to diagnose Parkinson's disease"			0.9999
True	2 (11%)	1 (14%)	
False	10 (53%)	4 (57%)	
Not Sure	7 (37%)	2 (29%)	
"Stress can worsen the condition"			0.2929
True	16 (84%)	4 (57%)	
False	0 (0%)	0 (0%)	
Not Sure	3 (16%)	3 (43%)	

Table 3. (Continued)

Question Item	**Under 20 n = 19**	**Over 20 n = 7**	**p-value**
"Exercise may slow the progression of Parkinson's disease"			0.9999
True	12 (63%)	4 (57%)	
False	2 (11%)	1 (14%)	
Not Sure	5 (26%)	2 (29%)	
"Parkinson's only affects old people"			0.9999
True	1 (5%)	0 (0%)	
False	18 (95%)	7 (100%)	
Not Sure	0 (0%)	0 (0%)	
"Men and women are equally as likely to be affected by Parkinson's"			0.1240
True	5 (26%)	1 (14%)	
False	6 (32%)	0 (0%)	
Not Sure	8 (42%)	6 (86%)	
"There is no correlation between Parkinson's and depression"			0.6576
True	0 (0%)	0 (0%)	
False	9 (47%)	2 (29%)	
Not Sure	10 (53%)	5 (71%)	
Knowledge Score			0.6679
Not Knowledgeable (0-4)	12 (63%)	5 (71%)	
Satisfactory (5-6)	4 (21%)	2 (29%)	
Knowledgeable (7-8)	3 (16%)	0 (0%)	
Mean ± SD	4.53 ± 1.50	3.71 ± 1.25	0.2106
Question Item	**Males n = 6**	**Females n = 20**	
"I believe I am knowledgeable about			0.7073
Parkinson's disease"	1 (17%)	3 (15%)	
Agree	1 (17%)	8 (40%)	
Disagree	4 (67%)	9 (45%)	
Neutral			
"The cause of Parkinson's disease is unknown"			0.6025
True	2 (33%)	6 (30%)	
False	2 (33%)	3 (15%)	
Not Sure	2 (33%)	11 (55%)	

Question Item	**Males** **n = 6**	**Females** **n = 20**	
"There is no cure to the disease, only treatments of symptoms"			0.9999
True	6 (100%)	17 (85%)	
False	0 (0%)	1 (5%)	
Not Sure	0 (0%)	2 (10%)	
"There is no specific test to diagnose Parkinson's disease"			0.8292
True	0 (0%)	3 (15%)	
False	4 (67%)	10 (50%)	
Not Sure	2 (33%)	7 (35%)	
"Stress can worsen the condition"			0.1119
True	3 (50%)	17 (85%)	
False	0 (0%)	0 (0%)	
Not Sure	3 (50%)	3 (15%)	
"Exercise may slow the progression of Parkinson's disease"			0.3819
True	3 (50%)	13 (65%)	
False	0 (0%)	3 (15%)	
Not Sure	3 (50%)	4 (20%)	
"Parkinson's only affects old people"			0.9999
True	0 (0%)	1 (5%)	
False	6 (100%)	19 (95%)	
Not Sure	0 (0%)	0 (0%)	
"Men and women are equally as likely to be affected by Parkinson's"			0.3395
True	0 (0%)	6 (30%)	
False	1 (17%)	5 (25%)	
Not Sure	5 (83%)	9 (45%)	
"There is no correlation between Parkinson's and depression"			0.6739
True	0 (0%)	0 (0%)	
False	3 (50%)	8 (40%)	
Not Sure	3 (50%)	12 (60%)	
Knowledge Score			0.9999
Not Knowledgeable (0-4)	4 (67%)	13 (65%)	
Satisfactory (5-6)	1 (17%)	5 (25%)	
Knowledgeable (7-8)	1 (17%)	2 (10%)	
Mean ± SD	4.00 ± 1.79	4.40 ± 1.39	0.5676

Table 3. (Continued)

Question Item	Affected n = 7	Unaffected n = 19	
"I believe I am knowledgeable about			0.0522
Parkinson's disease"	2 (29%)	2 (11%)	
Agree	0 (0%)	9 (47%)	
Disagree	5 (71%)	8 (42%)	
Neutral			
"The cause of Parkinson's disease is unknown"			0.0388
True	0 (0%)	8 (42%)	
False	3 (43%)	2 (11%)	
Not Sure	4 (57%)	9 (47%)	
"There is no cure to the disease, only treatments of symptoms"			0.9999
True	7 (100%)	16 (84%)	
False	0 (0%)	1 (5%)	
Not Sure	0 (0%)	2 (11%)	
"There is no specific test to diagnose Parkinson's disease"			0.8357
True	1 (14%)	2 (11%)	
False	3 (43%)	11 (58%)	
Not Sure	3 (43%)	6 (32%)	
"Stress can worsen the condition"			0.9999
True	5 (71%)	15 (79%)	
False	0 (0%)	0 (0%)	
Not Sure	2 (29%)	4 (21%)	
"Exercise may slow the progression of Parkinson's disease"			0.1271
True	3 (43%)	13 (68%)	
False	0 (0%)	3 (16%)	
Not Sure	4 (57%)	3 (16%)	
"Parkinson's only affects old people"			0.9999
True	0 (0%)	1 (5%)	
False	7 (100%)	18 (95%)	
Not Sure	0 (0%)	0 (0%)	

Question Item	Affected n = 7	Unaffected n = 19	
"Men and women are equally as likely to be affected by Parkinson's"			0.1240
True	1 (14%)	5 (26%)	
False	0 (0%)	6 (32%)	
Not Sure	6 (86%)	8 (42%)	
"There is no correlation between Parkinson's and depression"			0.4065
True	0 (0%)	0 (0%)	
False	4 (57%)	7 (37%)	
Not Sure	3 (43%)	12 (32%)	
Knowledge Score			0.6679
Not Knowledgeable (0-4)	5 (71%)	12 (32%)	
Satisfactory (5-6)	2 (29%)	4 (21%)	
Knowledgeable (7-8)	0 (0%)	3 (16%)	
Mean ± SD	3.86 ± 0.90	4.47 ± 1.61	0.3558
Question Item	**Less than 10 visits n = 4**	**More than 10 visits n = 3**	
"I believe I am knowledgeable about Parkinson's disease"			0.9999
Agree	1 (25%)	1 (33%)	
Disagree	0 (0%)	0 (0%)	
Neutral	3 (75%)	2 (67%)	
"The cause of Parkinson's disease is unknown"			0.9999
True	0 (0%)	0 (0%)	
False	2 (50%)	1 (33%)	
Not Sure	2 (50%)	2 (67%)	
"There is no cure to the disease, only treatments of symptoms"			0.9999
True	4 (100%)	3 (100%)	
False	0 (0%)	0 (0%)	
Not Sure	0 (0%)	0 (0%)	
"There is no specific test to diagnose Parkinson's disease"			0.9999
True	1 (25%)	0 (0%)	
False	1 (25%)	2 (67%)	
Not Sure	2 (50%)	1 (33%)	

Table 3. (Continued)

Question Item	Less than 10 visits n = 4	More than 10 visits n = 3	
"Stress can worsen the condition"			0.9999
True	3 (75%)	2 (67%)	
False	0 (0%)	0 (0%)	
Not Sure	1 (25%)	1 (33%)	
"Exercise may slow the progression of Parkinson's disease"			0.9999
True	2 (50%)	1 (33%)	
False	0 (0%)	0 (0%)	
Not Sure	2 (50%)	2 (67%)	
"Parkinson's only affects old people"			0.9999
True	0 (0%)	0 (0%)	
False	4 (100%)	3 (100%)	
Not Sure	0 (0%)	0 (0%)	
"Men and women are equally as likely to be affected by Parkinson's"			0.9999
True	1 (25%)	0 (0%)	
False	0 (0%)	0 (0%)	
Not Sure	3 (75%)	3 (100%)	
"There is no correlation between Parkinson's and depression"			0.4857
True	0 (0%)	0 (0%)	
False	3 (75%)	1 (33%)	
Not Sure	1 (25%)	2 (67%)	
Knowledge Score			0.4286
Not Knowledgeable (0-4)	2 (50%)	3 (100%)	
Satisfactory (5-6)	2 (50%)	0 (0%)	
Knowledgeable (7-8)	0 (0%)	0 (0%)	
Mean ± SD	4.25 ± 0.96	3.33 ± 0.58	0.2060

There seems to exist a difference in perceived awareness between those who have family members affected and unaffected by the disease, but there actually was no difference in overall awareness. Those who have a family member affected by the disease believe that they are more aware, with 29% compared to 11% claiming that they are knowledgeable about the disease ($p = 0.0522$). Those who were unaffected by the disease correctly answered at 42% of the time that the cause of the disease is unknown, compared to 0% of the time for those with a family member affected ($p = 0.0388$). 100% and 84% of those affected and unaffected, respectively, noted that there is no cure to the disease; 14% and 11% answered that there is no specific diagnostic test ($p = 0.8357$); 71% and 79% noted that stress can worsen the condition ($p = 0.9999$); 43% and 68% correctly responded that exercise may slow the progression ($p = 0.1271$); 100% and 95% noted that Parkinson's does not only affect old people ($p = 0.9999$); 14% and 26% incorrectly believed that men and women are equally as likely to be affected ($p = 0.1240$); 57% and 37% noted that there is a correlation between the disease and depression ($p = 0.4065$). Overall, there was no difference in the knowledge scores ($p = 0.6679$), and average scores for the two cohorts were 3.86 and 4.47 ($p = 0.3558$) (see Table 3).

The frequency of visits per year among those who have a family member affected by the disease did not seem to affect the perceived of actual awareness, as there was no difference noted. 25% and 33% of those who visited less than 10 and more than 10 times a year, respectively, believed that they were knowledgeable about the disease ($p = 0.9999$). There exists no difference in the individual knowledge questions ($p = 0.9999$ for all endpoints) - 50% and 33% incorrectly remarked that the cause of Parkinson's disease is known, 100% of both groups noted that there is no cure to the disease, 25% and 0% answered that there is no specific diagnostic test, 75% and 67% noted that stress can worsen the condition, 50% and 33% responded that exercise may slow the progression, 100% of both cohorts noted that it does not only affect old people, 25% and 0% incorrectly believed that is equally affects males and females, and 75% and 33% remarked that there is a correlation between Parkinson's and depression. Overall, 50% and 100% were not knowledgeable about the disease ($p = 0.4285$), and the mean scores were 4.25 and 3.33 out of 8 ($p = 0.2060$) (see Table 3).

Discussion

The results of this study are in line with those previously disclosed by Chow et al. about young adults in London, Canada (12) - young adults are adequately aware of the disease. While only 23% of young adults have family members affected by the disease and only 15% believe that they are knowledgeable, it turns out that 35% of the sample population is knowledgeable of the disease.

The results within also show that age, sex, familial ties and frequency of visitation to affected individuals do not affect the awareness level of the disease. It is especially disappointing that familial ties do not increase awareness, as it seems that caregivers have the same knowledgeability as individuals who are not exposed to the disease. Informational pamphlets could perhaps be distributed by healthcare professionals to caregivers to help increase the awareness level of these individuals, so that they can better care for their family members.

The overall 35% awareness level of the disease is lower than the 41% awareness level of young adults in London, Canada (12). Regardless of which region has a lower awareness level, the statistics suggest that there is plenty room for improvement. Educational programs can be established to help increase the awareness/knowledge of the general public. This increased awareness level could better establish the young adults to take care of the increasing prevalence of Parkinson's disease.

This study was not without limitations. Due to the nature of the study methodology (survey study), there exists a possibility of sample/response bias. Additionally, there was low statistical power in the subgroup analysis. Further studies should be conducted with larger sample sizes.

In conclusion, 35% of the young adults in Toronto, Canada, were aware of the disease. This number is higher than the 23% of young adults who have a family member affected by the disease and only 15% believe that they are knowledgeable, suggesting that young adults are adequately aware to take care of individuals with Parkinson's disease. The results also show that there exists variation in awareness by geographic region, and further studies should be conducted to investigate awareness in other regions.

REFERENCES

[1] Parkinson J. An essay on the shaking palsy. London: Whitingham Rowland, 1817.

[2] Global Parkinson's Disease Survey Steering Committee. Factors impacting on quality of life in Parkinson's disease: results from an international survey. Mov Disord 20-2;17:60-7.

[3] Chow R, Borean M, Hollenberg D, Merrick J. How aware/knowledgeable are young adults about Parkinson's disease? J Pain Manage 2019;12(1), in press.

[4] Polymeropoulos MH, Lavedan C, Leroy identified in families with Parkinson's disease. Science 1997;276:2045-7.

[5] Chaudhuri KR, Schapira AHV, Martinez-Martin P. The holistic management of Parkinson's using a novel non-motor symptom scale and questionnaire. Adv Clin Neurosci Rehabil 2004;4:20-4.

[6] Aarsland D, Larsen JP, Tandberg E, Laake K. Predictors of nursing home placement in Parkinson's disease: a population-based, prospective study. J Am Geriatr Soc 2000;48:938-42.

[7] Witjas T, Kaphan E, Azulay JP, Blin O, Ceccaldi M, Pouget J, et al. Nonmotor fluctuations in Parkinson's disease: frequent and disabling. Neurology 2002;59:408-13.

[8] Schrag A, Jahanshahi N, Quinn N. What contributes to quality of life in patients with Parkinson's disease? J Neurol Neurosurg Psychiatry 2000;69:308-12.

[9] Findley L, Aujla M, Bain PG, Baker M, Beech C, Bowman C, et al. Direct economic impact of Parkinson's disease: a research survey in the United Kingdom. Mov Disord 2003;18:1139-45.

[10] Pressley JC, Louis ED, Tang MX, Cote L, Cohen PD, Glied S, et al. The impact of comorbid disease and injuries on resource use and expenditures in Parkinsonism. Neurology 2003;60:87-93.

[11] Chow R, Viehweger J, Trasente V, Borean M, Hollenberg D, Lam M, et al. Awareness of Parkinson's disease among young adults in London, Canada. J Pain Manage 2019;12(1), in press.
[12] Chow R, Borean M, Hollenberg D. Awareness of Parkinson's disease: About the survey instrument. J Pain Manage 2019;12(1), in press.

In: Parkinson's Disease
Editors: Ronald Chow, et al.
ISBN: 978-1-53612-745-4

Chapter 5

AWARENESS OF PARKINSON'S DISEASE AMONG YOUNG ADULTS IN WATERLOO, CANADA

Jaclyn Viehweger, BMSc(C), Ronald Chow*, BMSc(C), Victoria Trasente, BA(C), Nathan Duarte, BASc(C), Michael Borean, BMSc(C), Drew Hollenberg, BMSc(C), Tharani Anpalagan, BMSc(C) and Anna Rzepka, BMSc(C)

Infinitas Research Group, London, Ontario, Canada

One of the best ways to improve care for patients affected by Parkinson's disease is to increase the knowledge and awareness of those who could potentially be caregivers for patients. The aim of this chapter was to evaluate the awareness of young adults in Waterloo, Ontario, Canada. A survey was circulated via social media outlets to young adults in Waterloo, Canada. The survey was voluntary. The consent form on the

* Correspondence: Ronald Chow BMSc(C), Infinitas Research Group, London, Ontario, Canada. Email: rchow48@uwo.ca.

first page acknowledged that there are no benefits/costs to participants, and required participants to consent to the study. The second page collected demographic information and the third page was used to determine the actual and perceived awareness of Parkinson's disease. A total of 19 consenting participants completed the survey. 58% of young adults are knowledgeable, which is higher than the statistics that 32% have a family member affected by the disease and that 26% perceived themselves to be knowledgeable. Rigorous educational programs can be developed to inform the community more about the disease, so that young adults can be better caregivers for those currently and who may in the future be affected by the disease.

INTRODUCTION

One of the best ways to improve care for patients affected by Parkinson's disease is to increase the knowledge and awareness of those who could potentially be caregivers for patients (1). By understanding the disease and the suffering that patients have to go through, such as the motor and nonmotor symptoms (i.e., tremor, muscle rigidity, postural instability, depression), caregivers can consequently provide more individualized care (2-7). Such individualized care is one of the best options for such a disease, especially considering that there does not exist a cure to the treatment today (1).

Two studies have been conducted to look into the awareness levels of young adults with respect to Parkinson's disease - the original study conducted by Chow et al. in London, Canada, and a second (follow-up) study published by Ho et al. in Toronto, Canada (8-9). Both studies circulated a survey to young adults in their respective communities (10). Chow et al. (8) noted that 41% of young adults believed they were knowledgeable, which is in excess of the statistic that only 27% have a family member affected by the disease. Both of these statistics noted by Chow et al. are lower than that actual awareness level, where 54% of young adults are aware of the disease (8).

The trend that young adults are adequately aware to take care of their family members was similarly noted by Ho et al. (9) in Toronto. From the 26 participants they surveyed, 35% of young adults were aware of the disease - higher than both the perceived awareness (15%) and the percentage of individuals who have a family member affected by the disease (23%) (9).

While these studies support the conclusion that young adults are adequately aware of Parkinson's disease, the conglomerate sample size of these two studies are small. The two studies also show that there exists variation between geographic locations. The aim of this study was to re-evaluate the awareness of young adults, but in Waterloo, Ontario, Canada.

OUR STUDY

A survey was circulated via social media outlets to young adults in Waterloo, Canada. The survey was voluntary. The consent form on the first page acknowledged that there are no benefits/costs to participants, and required participants to consent to the study. The second page collected demographic information and the third page was used to determine the actual and perceived awareness of Parkinson's disease (10).

Descriptive statistics were used to share participant demographics, and the number of correct/incorrect answers. Fisher exact tests were used to determine whether there was a difference in categorical questions between age groups (under and over 20 years old), gender groups (males and females), familial ties (affected and not affected by Parkinson's disease) and the frequency of visiting their family members (less than and over 10 visits a year). ANOVA procedures compared the average number of correct answers between the subgroups. All analyses were conducted using the Statistical Analysis Software (SAS Version 9.4 for Windows) (10).

Our findings

A total of 19 consenting participants completed the survey. 12 (63%) respondents were between 18 and 19 years old, 3 (16%) were between 20 and 22 years old and 4 (21%) were over 22 years old. 84% reported that they were female, and 16% were male. 32% remarked that to their knowledge, they have a family member affected by Parkinson's disease. Among those 32%, 50% visited their family member less than 3 times a year and 50% visited their family member between 10 and 20 times a year (see Table 1).

Table 1. Demographics

Demographic	**n = 19**
Age Group	
Under 18 years old	0 (0%)
18-19 years old	12 (63%)
20-22 years old	3 (16%)
Over 22 years old	4 (21%)
Sex	
Male	3 (16%)
Female	16 (84%)
Prefer not to say	0 (0%)
Family member affected by Parkinson's disease	
Yes	6 (32%)
No	13 (68%)
Number of visits to Parkinson's family member a year (n=6)	
Less than 3	3 (50%)
3-10	0 (0%)
10-20	3 (50%)
20+	0 (0%)

Table 2. Perceived and actual knowledge

Question Item	n = 19
"I believe I am knowledgeable about Parkinson's disease"	
Agree	5 (26%)
Disagree	6 (32%)
Neutral	8 (42%)
"The cause of Parkinson's disease is unknown"	
True	8 (42%)
False	1 (5%)
Not Sure	10 (53%)
"There is no cure to the disease, only treatments of symptoms"	
True	16 (84%)
False	1 (5%)
Not Sure	2 (11%)
"There is no specific test to diagnose Parkinson's disease"	
True	3 (16%)
False	8 (42%)
Not Sure	8 (42%)
"Stress can worsen the condition"	
True	13 (68%)
False	1 (5%)
Not Sure	5 (26%)
"Exercise may slow the progression of Parkinson's disease"	
True	9 (47%)
False	1 (5%)
Not Sure	9 (47%)
"Parkinson's only affects old people"	
True	1 (5%)
False	17 (90%)
Not Sure	1 (5%)
"Men and women are equally as likely to be affected by Parkinson's"	
True	3 (16%)
False	9 (47%)
Not Sure	7 (37%)

Table 2. (Continued)

Question Item	n = 19
"There is no correlation between Parkinson's and depression"	
True	2 (10%)
False	11 (58%)
Not Sure	6 (32%)
Knowledge Score	
Not Knowledgeable (0-4)	8 (42%)
Satisfactory (5-6)	8 (42%)
Knowledgeable (7-8)	3 (16%)
Mean ± SD	4.53 ± 1.81

26% of respondents believed that they were knowledgeable about Parkinson's disease. 42% correctly answered that there is no known cause to Parkinson's disease; 84% noted that there is no cure to the disease; 16% indicated that there is no specific diagnostic test; 68% reported that stress can worsen the condition; 47% answered that exercise may slow the progression; 90% remarked that the disease does not only affect old people; 47% answered that men and women are not equally as likely to be affected; 58% responded that there is a correlation between Parkinson's disease and depression. 16% were considered knowledgeable, and 42% were deemed as having satisfactory knowledge; the average score was 4.53 out of 8 (see Table 2).

There exists a difference in perceived awareness between age cohorts, but no difference in actual awareness. 29% of the older group (over 20 years old) believe that they are knowledgeable about Parkinson's disease, while 25% of the younger group similarly noted such an answer ($p=0.0393$). Those older than 20 years old were more knowledgeable with respect to the first question - 86% compared to 17% correctly answered that the cause of the disease is unknown ($p=0.0128$). 83% and 86% of the two groups, respectively, answered that there is no cure to the disease (p=0.2817); 33% and 57% incorrectly responded that there is a diagnostic test (p=0.3932); 75% and 57% reported that stress can worsen the condition (p=0.5743); 42% and 57% remarked that exercise may slow the progression of the disease (p=0.9999); 83% and 100% noted that it does not only affect old people (p=0.9999); 17% and 14% inaccurately answered that men and women are equally as likely to be affected by the disease (p=0.8250); 50% and 71% noted that there is a correlation between Parkinson's and depression (p=0.4040). 42% and 43% noted that participants had satisfactory knowledge (p=0.5799), and the two cohorts had average scores of 4.17 and 5.14, respectively (p=0.2708) (see Table 3).

Table 3. Perceived and actual knowledge - by subgroups

Question Item	**Under 20** **n = 12**	**Over 20** **n = 7**	**p-value**
"I believe I am knowledgeable about Parkinson's disease"			0.0393
Agree	3 (25%)	2 (29%)	
Disagree	6 (50%)	0 (0%)	
Neutral	3 (25%)	5 (71%)	
"The cause of Parkinson's disease is unknown"			0.0128
True	2 (17%)	6 (86%)	
False	1 (8%)	0 (0%)	
Not Sure	9 (75%)	1 (14%)	
"There is no cure to the disease, only treatments of symptoms"			0.2817
True	10 (83%)	6 (86%)	
False	0 (0%)	1 (14%)	
Not Sure	2 (17%)	0 (0%)	

Table 3. (Continued)

Question Item	Under 20 n = 12	Over 20 n = 7	p-value
"There is no specific test to diagnose Parkinson's disease"			0.3932
True	3 (25%)	0 (0%)	
False	4 (33%)	4 (57%)	
Not Sure	5 (42%)	3 (43%)	
"Stress can worsen the condition"			0.5743
True	9 (75%)	4 (57%)	
False	0 (0%)	1 (14%)	
Not Sure	3 (25%)	2 (29%)	
"Exercise may slow the progression of Parkinson's disease"			0.9999
True	5 (42%)	4 (57%)	
False	1 (8%)	0 (0%)	
Not Sure	6 (50%)	3 (43%)	
"Parkinson's only affects old people"			0.9999
True	1 (8%)	0 (0%)	
False	10 (83%)	7 (100%)	
Not Sure	1 (8%)	0 (0%)	
"Men and women are equally as likely to be affected by Parkinson's"			0.8250
True	2 (17%)	1 (14%)	
False	5 (42%)	4 (57%)	
Not Sure	5 (42%)	2 (29%)	
"There is no correlation between Parkinson's and depression"			0.4040
True	1 (8%)	1 (14%)	
False	6 (50%)	5 (71%)	
Not Sure	5 (42%)	1 (14%)	
Knowledge Score			
Not Knowledgeable (0-4)	6 (50%)	2 (29%)	0.5799
Satisfactory (5-6)	5 (42%)	3 (43%)	
Knowledgeable (7-8)	1 (8%)	2 (29%)	
Mean ± SD	4.17 ± 1.85	5.14 ± 1.68	0.2708

Question Item	**Males** **n = 3**	**Females** **n = 16**	
"I believe I am knowledgeable about Parkinson's disease"			0.9999
Agree	1 (33%)	4 (25%)	
Disagree	1 (33%)	5 (31%)	
Neutral	1 (33%)	7 (44%)	
"The cause of Parkinson's disease is unknown"			0.9999
True	1 (33%)	7 (44%)	
False	0 (0%)	1 (6%)	
Not Sure	2 (66%)	8 (50%)	
"There is no cure to the disease, only treatments of symptoms"			0.9999
True	3 (100%)	13 (81%)	
False	0 (0%)	1 (6%)	
Not Sure	0 (0%)	2 (13%)	
"There is no specific test to diagnose Parkinson's disease"			0.3395
True	1 (33%)	2 (13%)	
False	2 (66%)	6 (38%)	
Not Sure	0 (0%)	8 (50%)	
"Stress can worsen the condition"			0.5975
True	3 (100%)	10 (63%)	
False	0 (0%)	1 (6%)	
Not Sure	0 (0%)	5 (31%)	
"Exercise may slow the progression of Parkinson's disease"			0.3313
True	3 (100%)	6 (38%)	
False	0 (0%)	1 (6%)	
Not Sure	0 (0%)	9 (56%)	
"Parkinson's only affects old people"			0.2982
True	1 (33%)	0 (0%)	
False	2 (66%)	15 (94%)	
Not Sure	0 (0%)	1 (6%)	

Table 3. (Continued)

Question Item	Males n = 3	Females n = 16	
"Men and women are equally as likely to be affected by Parkinson's"			0.7399
True	1 (33%)	2 (13%)	
False	1 (33%)	8 (50%)	
Not Sure	1 (33%)	6 (38%)	
"There is no correlation between Parkinson's and depression"			0.1827
True	1 (33%)	1 (6%)	
False	2 (66%)	9 (56%)	
Not Sure	0 (0%)	6 (38%)	
Knowledge Score			
Not Knowledgeable (0-4)	1 (33%)	7 (44%)	0.5377
Satisfactory (5-6)	1 (33%)	7 (44%)	
Knowledgeable (7-8)	1 (33%)	2 (13%)	
Mean ± SD	5.33 ± 1.53	4.38 ± 1.86	0.4193
Question Item	**Affected n = 6**	**Unaffected n = 13**	
"I believe I am knowledgeable about Parkinson's disease"			0.4634
Agree	1 (17%)	4 (31%)	
Disagree	1 (17%)	5 (38%)	
Neutral	4 (66%)	4 (31%)	
"The cause of Parkinson's disease is unknown"			0.9999
True	3 (50%)	5 (38%)	
False	0 (0%)	1 (8%)	
Not Sure	3 (50%)	7 (54%)	
"There is no cure to the disease, only treatments of symptoms"			0.6780
True	6 (100%)	10 (77%)	
False	0 (0%)	1 (8%)	
Not Sure	0 (0%)	2 (15%)	

Question Item	**Affected n = 6**	**Unaffected n = 13**	
"There is no specific test to diagnose Parkinson's disease"			0.1827
True	2 (33%)	1 (8%)	
False	1 (17%)	7 (54%)	
Not Sure	3 (50%)	5 (38%)	
"Stress can worsen the condition"			0.7365
True	5 (83%)	8 (62%)	
False	0 (0%)	1 (8%)	
Not Sure	1 (17%)	4 (31%)	
"Exercise may slow the progression of Parkinson's disease"			0.4056
True	3 (50%)	6 (46%)	
False	1 (17%)	0 (0%)	
Not Sure	2 (33%)	7 (54%)	
"Parkinson's only affects old people"			0.5439
True	1 (17%)	0 (0%)	
False	5 (83%)	12 (92%)	
Not Sure	0 (0%)	1 (8%)	
"Men and women are equally as likely to be affected by Parkinson's"			0.0650
True	2 (33%)	1 (8%)	
False	4 (66%)	5 (38%)	
Not Sure	0 (0%)	7 (54%)	
"There is no correlation between Parkinson's and depression"			0.6351
True	1 (17%)	1 (8%)	
False	4 (66%)	7 (54%)	
Not Sure	1 (17%)	5 (38%)	
Knowledge Score			
Not Knowledgeable (0-4)	1 (17%)	7 (54%)	0.3065
Satisfactory (5-6)	4 (66%)	4 (31%)	
Knowledgeable (7-8)	1 (17%)	2 (15%)	
Mean ± SD	5.33 ± 1.03	4.15 ± 1.99	0.1927

Table 3. (Continued)

Question Item	**Less than 10 visits n = 3**	**More than 10 visits n = 3**	
"I believe I am knowledgeable about Parkinson's disease"			0.4000
Agree	1 (33%)	0 (0%)	
Disagree	1 (33%)	0 (0%)	
Neutral	1 (33%)	3 (100%)	
"The cause of Parkinson's disease is unknown"			0.9999
True	2 (66%)	1 (33%)	
False	0 (0%)	0 (0%)	
Not Sure	1 (33%)	2 (67%)	
"There is no cure to the disease, only treatments of symptoms"			0.9999
True	3 (100%)	3 (100%)	
False	0 (0%)	0 (0%)	
Not Sure	0 (0%)	0 (0%)	
"There is no specific test to diagnose Parkinson's disease"			0.1000
True	2 (66%)	0 (0%)	
False	1 (33%)	0 (0%)	
Not Sure	0 (0%)	3 (100%)	
"Stress can worsen the condition"			0.9999
True	3 (100%)	2 (66%)	
False	0 (0%)	0 (0%)	
Not Sure	0 (0%)	1 (33%)	
"Exercise may slow the progression of Parkinson's disease"			0.4000
True	2 (66%)	1 (33%)	
False	1 (33%)	0 (0%)	
Not Sure	0 (0%)	2 (66%)	

Question Item	Less than 10 visits n = 3	More than 10 visits n = 3	
"Parkinson's only affects old people"			0.9999
True	1 (33%)	0 (0%)	
False	2 (66%)	3 (100%)	
Not Sure	0 (0%)	0 (0%)	
"Men and women are equally as likely to be affected by Parkinson's"			0.4000
True	2 (66%)	0 (0%)	
False	1 (33%)	3 (100%)	
Not Sure	0 (0%)	0 (0%)	
"There is no correlation between Parkinson's and depression"			0.9999
True	1 (33%)	0 (0%)	
False	2 (66%)	2 (66%)	
Not Sure	0 (0%)	1 (33%)	
Knowledge Score			
Not Knowledgeable (0-4)	1 (33%)	0 (0%)	0.4000
Satisfactory (5-6)	1 (33%)	3 (100%)	
Knowledgeable (7-8)	1 (33%)	0 (0%)	
Mean ± SD	5.67 ± 1.53	5.00 ± 0.00	0.4904

Perceived and actual awareness of males and females were similar. 33% and 25% of males and females, respectively, believed they are knowledgeable about the disease (p=0.9999). 33% and 44% answered that the cause of the disease is unknown (p=0.9999); 100% and 81% remarked that there is no cure to the disease (p=0.9999); 33% and 13% noted that there is no specific test to the disease (p=0.3395); the fact that stress can worsen the condition was indicated by 100% and 63% (p=0.5975); 100% and 38% answered that exercise may slow the progression of the disease (p=0.3313). 66% and 94% responded that Parkinson's does not only affect old people (p=0.2982); 33% and 50% answered that men and women are not equally as likely to be affected by the disease (p=0.7399); 66% and 56% concluded that there is a correlation between the disease and depression (p=0.1827). 33% and 44% of the two groups, respectively, had a satisfactory knowledge score (p=0.5377). The two sex cohorts had mean scores of 5.33 and 4.38, respectively (p=0.4193) (see table 3).

When subgroup analysis was conducted between affected and unaffected individuals, there existed no difference in any questions with regards to awareness. 17% of those affected and 31% of those unaffected reported that they are knowledgeable about the disease (p=0.4634). 50% and 38% remarked that the cause of the disease is unknown (p=0.9999); 100% and 77% answered that there is no cure to the disease (p=0.6780); 33% and 8% noted that there is no diagnostic test (p=0.1827); 83% and 62% concluded that stress can worsen the condition (p=0.7365). The fact that exercise may slow the progression was correctly noted by 50% and 46% (p=0.4056); 83% and 92% noted that Parkinson's does not only affect old people (p=0.5439); 66% and 38% indicated that men and women are not equally as affected by the disease (p=0.0650); 66% and 54% answered that there is a correlation between the disease and depression (p=0.6351). The average knowledge scores were 5.33 and 4.15, respectively (p=0.1927), with 17% and 54% deemed not knowledgeable (p=0.3065) (see table 3).

There also existed no difference among those who are affected by the disease, between those who frequently and do not frequently visit their afflicted family members. 33% compared to 0% noted that they are knowledgeable about the disease (p=0.4000). 66% and 33% remarked that the cause of the disease is unknown (p=0.9999); 100% of both cohorts reported that there is no cure to the disease (p=0.9999); 66% and 0% answered that there is no diagnostic test (p=0.1000); 100% and 66% indicated that stress can worsen the condition (p=0.9999); 66% and 33% noted that exercise may slow the progression of the disease; 33% and 0% reported that it does not only affect old people (p=0.9999); 33% and 100% concluded that the two sexes are not equally as likely to be affected by the disease (p=0.4000); 66% of both cohorts noted that there is a correlation between the disease and depression (p=0.9999). 33% and 0% of the groups had satisfactory knowledge (p=0.4000), and had average scores of 5.67 and 5.00, respectively (p=0.4904) (see Table 3).

DISCUSSION

58% of young adults have adequate knowledge of the disease, as determined by this survey. 32% of family members are affected by the disease and 26% perceived themselves to be knowledgeable; both statistics are lower than the actual awareness level, which is encouraging to note that young adults are adequately aware.

The reported awareness level of young adults in Waterloo is higher than those reported by Chow et al. in London (54%) and Ho et al. in Toronto (35%). However, no analysis was conducted to determine whether such a difference is statistically significant. Especially given that this sample size is smaller than the other two studies, such an awareness level could simply be an anomaly; what is for certain is that there seems to exist variation by geographic location.

The subgroup analysis also revealed that the awareness /knowledgeability level of young adults does not differ depending on demographics (sex and age) or personal history. This seems to indicate that having a family member affected by the disease does not increase the awareness of the disease. Hence, it seems that the only way to logically increase awareness is to develop rigorous educational programs to inform the community about the disease, so that young adults can ultimately become excellent caregivers for this disease that will become more prevalent in the future.

This study had its limitations. As a result of study design (survey), there is the possibility of a sampling/response bias. The small sample size also did not allow high statistical power for subgroup analyses between sex and those members afflicted by the disease.

In conclusion, 58% of young adults are knowledgeable, which is higher than the statistics that 32% have a family member affected by the disease and that 26% perceived themselves to be knowledgeable. Rigorous educational programs can be developed to inform the community more about the disease, so that young adults can be better caregivers for those currently and who may in the future be affected by the disease.

REFERENCES

[1] Chow R, Borean M, Hollenberg D, Merrick J. How aware/knowledgeable are young adults about Parkinson's disease? J Pain Manage 2019;12(1), in press.

[2] Parkinson J. An essay on the shaking palsy. London: Whitingham Rowland, 1817.

[3] Global Parkinson's Disease Survey Steering Committee. Factors impacting on quality of life in Parkinson's disease: results from an international survey. Mov Disord 20-2;17:60-7.

[4] Polymeropoulos MH, Lavedan C, Leroy E, Ide SE, Dehejia A, Dutra A, et al. Mutation in the α-Synuclein Gene Identified in Families with Parkinson's Disease. Science 1997;276:2045-7.

[5] Chaudhuri KR, Schapira AHV, Martinez-Martin P. The holistic management of Parkinson's using a novel non-motor symptom scale and questionnaire. Adv Clin Neurosci Rehabil 2004;4:20-4.

[6] Aarsland D, Larsen JP, Tandberg E, Laake K. Predictors of nursing home placement in Parkinson's disease: a population-based, prospective study. J Am Geriatr Soc 2000;48:938-42.

[7] Witjas T, Kaphan E, Azulay JP, Blin O, Ceccaldi M, Pouget J, et al. Nonmotor fluctuations in Parkinson's disease: frequent and disabling. Neurology 2002;59:408-13.

[8] Chow R, Viehweger J, Trasente V, Borean M, Hollenberg D, Lam M, et al. Awareness of Parkinson's disease among young adults in London, Canada. J Pain Manage 2019;12(1), in press.

[9] Ho S, Viehweger J, Trasente V, Ho C, Ng W, Wong M, et al. Awareness of Parkinson's disease among young adults in Toronto, Canada. J Pain Manage 2019;12(1), in press.

[10] Chow R, Borean M, Hollenberg D. Awareness of Parkinson's disease: About the survey instrument. J Pain Manage 2019;12(1), in press.

In: Parkinson's Disease
Editors: Ronald Chow, et al.
ISBN: 978-1-53612-745-4

Chapter 6

AWARENESS OF PARKINSON'S DISEASE AMONG YOUNG ADULTS IN HALIFAX, CANADA

Stephanie Ho, Jaclyn Viehweger, BMSc(C), Victoria Trasente, BA(C), Michael Borean, BMSc(C), Drew Hollenberg, BMSc(C), Tyler Ferguson, BComm(C), Tharani Anpalagan, BMSc(C), Anna Rzepka, BMSc(C) and Ronald Chow*, BMSc(C)
Infinitas Research Group, London, Ontario, Canada

The objective of this chapter was to evaluate the awareness of Parkinson's disease amongst young adults in Halifax, Canada. A questionnaire was sent out via social media outlets. The survey was

* Correspondence: Ronald Chow BMSc(C), Infinitas Research Group, London, Ontario, Canada. Email: rchow48@uwo.ca.

voluntary. The consent form on the first page acknowledged that there are no benefits/costs to participants, and required participants to consent to the study. The second page collected demographic information and the third page was used to determine the actual and perceived awareness of Parkinson's disease. A total of 15 individuals consented and completed the study. 80% were between 18 and 19 years old, 1 was between 20 and 22 years old, and 2 were over 22 years old. All respondents were female, and only 1 had a family member affected by Parkinson's, who she visits more than 20 times a year. 40% of participants were knowledgeable about the disease, which is higher than the statistics that 27% perceived themselves to be knowledgeable and 7% had a family member affected by the disease. In support of prior studies, education programs should be developed to increase awareness across the population.

Introduction

Three studies have investigated into whether young adults are aware of Parkinson's disease (1-3). This topic is very important, as awareness is the best way to increase quality of care for patients affected by the disease that manifests itself in debilitating motor and nonmotor symptoms (4-9). Increasing the awareness will hopefully allow for young adults to better understand the symptoms experienced by patients (i.e., depression, tremor, muscle rigidity) for a disease that does not have a cure (4-10).

The original study conducted in London, Canada by Chow et al. (1) noted that 54% of young adults were knowledgeable about the disease. 41% of those respondents believed they were knowledgeable, and 27% had family members affected by the disease. These statistics suggest that young adults are adequately aware to take care of their family members affected by the disease (1).

Two other studies have verified the trend revealed in the original study (2-3). A study from Toronto concluded that 35% of the population was knowledgeable, which was higher than the perceived awareness level of 15% and the 23% of individuals affected by the disease (2). Viehweger et al. published a study conducted among young adults in Waterloo, Canada, and observed awareness level to be at 58%, perceived awareness level to be 26%, and also that 32% of participants have a family member suffering from the disease (3).

While all three studies have verified the trend that young adults seem to be adequately aware of the disease, the studies show that there are variations between different demographic regions. This may be a result of the differing prevalence of the disease in different populations, or perhaps a result of different emphasis of the disease within their local communities. It's also important to note that all three studies were conducted within a single province of Canada; it would be interesting to note whether greater variation is noted in another Canadian province. Our objective was to evaluate the awareness of young adults in Halifax, Canada.

QUESTIONNAIRE

A questionnaire was sent out via social media outlets to young adults in Halifax, Canada. The survey was voluntary. The consent form on the first page acknowledged that there are no benefits/costs to participants, and required participants to consent to the study. The second page collected demographic information and the third page was used to determine the actual and perceived awareness of Parkinson's disease (11).

Descriptive statistics were used to disclose participant demographics, and the number of correct/incorrect answers. Fisher exact tests were used to determine whether there was a difference in categorical questions between age groups (under and over 20 years old), gender groups (males and females), familial ties (affected and not affected by Parkinson's disease) and the frequency of visiting their family members (less than and over 10 visits a year). ANOVA procedures compared the average number of correct answers between the subgroups. All analyses were conducted using the Statistical Analysis Software (SAS Version 9.4 for Windows) (11).

FINDINGS

A total of 15 individuals consented and completed the study. 80% were between 18 and 19 years old, 1 was between 20 and 22 years old, and 2 were over 22 years old. All respondents were female, and only 1 had a family member affected by Parkinson's, who she visits more than 20 times a year (see Table 1).

Table 1. Demographics

Demographic	**n = 15**
Age Group	
Under 18 years old	0 (0%)
18-19 years old	12 (80%)
20-22 years old	1 (7%)
Over 22 years old	2 (13%)
Sex	
Male	0 (0%)
Female	15 (100%)
Prefer not to say	0 (0%)
Family member affected by Parkinson's disease	
Yes	1 (7%)
No	14 (93%)
Number of visits to Parkinson's family member a year (n= 1)	
Less than 3	0 (0%)
3-10	0 (0%)
10-20	0 (0%)
20+	1 (100%)

Table 2. Perceived and actual knowledge

Question Item	**n = 15**
"I believe I am knowledgeable about Parkinson's disease"	
Agree	4 (27%)
Disagree	6 (40%)
Neutral	5 (33%)
"The cause of Parkinson's disease is unknown"	
True	6 (40%)
False	0 (0%)
Not Sure	9 (60%)
"There is no cure to the disease, only treatments of symptoms"	
True	11 (73%)
False	1 (6%)
Not Sure	3 (20%)
"There is no specific test to diagnose Parkinson's disease"	
True	2 (13%)
False	7 (47%)
Not Sure	6 (40%)
"Stress can worsen the condition"	
True	6 (40%)
False	2 (13%)
Not Sure	7 (47%)
"Exercise may slow the progression of Parkinson's disease"	
True	6 (40%)
False	1 (6%)
Not Sure	8 (53%)
"Parkinson's only affects old people"	
True	0 (0%)
False	14 (93%)
Not Sure	1 (6%)
"Men and women are equally as likely to be affected by Parkinson's"	
True	2 (13%)
False	4 (27%)
Not Sure	9 (60%)

Table 2. (Continued)

Question Item	n = 15
"There is no correlation between Parkinson's and depression"	
True	1 (6%)
False	9 (60%)
Not Sure	5 (33%)
Knowledge Score	
Not Knowledgeable (0-4)	9 (60%)
Satisfactory (5-6)	5 (33%)
Knowledgeable (7-8)	1 (6%)
Mean ± SD	3.87 ± 1.88

27% of respondents believed they were knowledgeable about Parkinson's disease. 40% correctly noted that the cause of Parkinson's disease is unknown, and 73% indicated that there is no cure to the disease. 13% rightfully noted that there is no specific diagnostic test, 40% concluded that stress can worsen the condition, and 40% responded that exercise may slow the progression fo the disease. All but one respondent (93%) noted that Parkinson's does not only affect old people, 27% remarked that men and women are not equally as likely to be affected by the disease, and 60% noted that there is a correlation between Parkinson's and depression. Overall, 60% were not knowledgeable with respect to Parkinson's disease, and the average score was 3.87 out of 8 (see Table 2).

There seems to exist a difference in perceived knowledge with respect to Parkinson's between the age cohorts, but in reality there exists none. All of those over 20 years old reserved judgement about their knowledge, compared to only 17% of those under 20 years old (p=0.0308). 33% and 66% of the cohorts, respectively, noted that the cause of the disease is unknown (p=0.5253); 75% and 66% noted that there is no cure to the disease (p=0.2747); 17% and 0% reported that there is no specific diagnostic test (p=0.7231); 42% and 33% indicated that stress can worsen the condition (p=0.4923); 42% and 33% also answered that exercise may slow the progression of the disease (p=0.9999); 92% and 100% concluded that men and women are not equally as likely to be affected by the disease (p=0.3407); 58% and 66% noted that there is a correlation between Parkinson's and depression (p=0.1231). There existed no difference in overall scores, with the average scores being 3.92 and 3.67, respectively (p=0.8462), and 58% and 66% were not knowledgeable (p=0.9999) (see Table 3).

Table 3. Perceived and actual knowledge - by subgroups

Question Item	**Under 20 n = 12**	**Over 20 n = 3**	**p-value**
"I believe I am knowledgeable about Parkinson's disease"			0.0308
Agree	4 (33%)	0 (0%)	
Disagree	6 (50%)	0 (0%)	
Neutral	2 (17%)	3 (100%)	
"The cause of Parkinson's disease is unknown"			0.5253
True	4 (33%)	2 (66%)	
False	0 (0%)	0 (0%)	
Not Sure	8 (67%)	1 (33%)	
"There is no cure to the disease, only treatments of symptoms"			0.2747
True	9 (75%)	2 (66%)	
False	0 (0%)	1 (33%)	
Not Sure	3 (25%)	0 (0%)	
"There is no specific test to diagnose Parkinson's disease"			0.7231
True	2 (17%)	0 (0%)	
False	6 (50%)	1 (33%)	
Not Sure	4 (33%)	2 (66%)	

Table 3. (Continued)

Question Item	**Under 20** **n = 12**	**Over 20** **n = 3**	**p-value**
"Stress can worsen the condition"			0.4923
True	5 (42%)	1 (33%)	
False	1 (7%)	1 (33%)	
Not Sure	6 (50%)	1 (33%)	
"Exercise may slow the progression of Parkinson's disease"			0.9999
True	5 (42%)	1 (33%)	
False	1 (7%)	0 (0%)	
Not Sure	6 (50%)	2 (66%)	
"Parkinson's only affects old people"			0.9999
True	0 (0%)	0 (0%)	
False	11 (92%)	3 (100%)	
Not Sure	1 (7%)	0 (0%)	
"Men and women are equally as likely to be affected by Parkinson's"			0.3407
True	1 (7%)	1 (33%)	
False	4 (33%)	0 (0%)	
Not Sure	7 (58%)	2 (66%)	
"There is no correlation between Parkinson's and depression"			0.1231
True	0 (0%)	1 (33%)	
False	7 (58%)	2 (66%)	
Not Sure	5 (42%)	0 (0%)	
Knowledge Score			
Not Knowledgeable (0-4)	7 (58%)	2 (66%)	0.9999
Satisfactory (5-6)	4 (33%)	1 (33%)	
Knowledgeable (7-8)	1 (7%)	0 (0%)	
Mean ± SD	3.92 ± 2.07	3.67 ± 1.15	0.8462

DISCUSSION

This study reports that 40% of participants were knowledgeable about the disease. This statistic is higher than both the perceived level of knowledge (27% believed they were knowledgeable) and the percentage of participants with a family member affected by the disease (7%). The results within are encouraging and indicate that young adults are adequately aware of the disease; it also aligns with other previously published studies of this nature (1-3).

This study did not note any differences in responses between cohorts. Although there was not enough data to analyze the data by sex and by familial ties, the results (albeit small sample size) still support prior conclusions that age does not seem to be a predictor for knowledge level. In support of prior studies, education programs should be developed to increase awareness across the population.

This study was not without limitations. As it is a survey study, there exists the possibility of a response/sampling bias. Additionally, this study has the smallest sample size of any study done to date and consequently did not allow for certain subgroup analyses to be even conducted.

In conclusion, 40% of participants were knowledgeable about the disease, which is higher than the statistics that 27% perceived themselves to be knowledgeable and 7% had a family member affected by the disease. In support of prior studies, education programs should be developed to increase awareness across the population.

REFERENCES

[1] Chow R, Viehweger J, Trasente V, Borean M, Hollenberg D, Lam M, et al. Awareness of Parkinson's disease among young adults in London, Canada. J Pain Manage 2019;12(1), in press.

[2] Ho S, Viehweger J, Trasente V, Ho C, Ng W, Wong M et al. Awareness of Parkinson's disease among young adults in Toronto, Canada. J Pain Manage 2019;12(1), in press.

[3] Viehweger J, Chow R, Trasente V, Duarte N, Borean M, Hollenberg D et al. Awareness of Parkinson's disease among young adults in Waterloo, Canada. J Pain Manage 2019;12(1), in press.

[4] Parkinson J. An essay on the shaking palsy. London: Whitingham Rowland, 1817.

[5] Global Parkinson's Disease Survey Steering Committee. Factors impacting on quality of life in Parkinson's disease: results from an international survey. Mov Disord 20-2;17:60-7.

[6] Polymeropoulos MH, Lavedan C, Leroy E, Ide SE, Dehejia A, Dutra A, et al. Mutation in the α-Synuclein Gene Identified in Families with Parkinson's Disease. Science 1997;276:2045-7.

[7] Chaudhuri KR, Schapira AHV, Martinez-Martin P. The holistic management of Parkinson's using a novel non-motor symptom scale and questionnaire. Adv Clin Neurosci Rehabil 2004;4:20-4.

[8] Aarsland D, Larsen JP, Tandberg E, Laake K. Predictors of nursing home placement in Parkinson's disease: a population-based, prospective study. J Am Geriatr Soc 2000;48:938-42.

[9] Witjas T, Kaphan E, Azulay JP, Blin O, Ceccaldi M, Pouget J, et al. Nonmotor fluctuations in Parkinson's disease: Frequent and disabling. Neurology 2002;59:408-13.

[10] Chow R, Borean M, Hollenberg D, Merrick J. How aware/knowledgeable are young adults about Parkinson's disease? J Pain Manage 2019;12(1), in press.

[11] Chow R, Borean M, Hollenberg D. Awareness of Parkinson's disease: About the survey instrument. J Pain Manage 2019;12(1), in press.

In: Parkinson's Disease
Editors: Ronald Chow, et al.
ISBN: 978-1-53612-745-4

Chapter 7

AWARENESS OF PARKINSON'S DISEASE AMONG YOUNG ADULTS IN KINGSTON, CANADA

Michael Borean, BMSc(C), Tharani Anpalagan, BMSc(C), Jaclyn Viehweger, BMSc(C), Logan Midroni, BSc(C), Cooper Midroni, BASc(C), Drew Hollenberg, BMSc(C), Victoria Trasente, BA(C), Anna Rzepka, BMSc(C), and Ronald Chow*, BMSc(C)
Infinitas Research Group, London, Ontario, Canada

The purpose of this chapter is to learn about the awareness of Parkinson's disease in the young adults of Kingston, Canada. A questionnaire was circulated to this population in the specified area through social media platforms. Fisher exact tests were applied between age groups (under and

* Correspondence: Ronald Chow BMSc(C), Infinitas Research Group, London, Ontario, Canada. Email: rchow48@uwo.ca.

over 20 year olds), gender groups (males and females), family history with the disease (affected and not affected by Parkinson's disease) and the frequency of visiting their family members (less than and over 10 visits a year). ANOVA procedures were used to evaluate the average number of correct answers between the subgroups. The survey was completed by 24 people, of which 33% believed they were knowledgeable about the disease. This value is lower than the 39% of respondents who had an adequate knowledge of the disease, indicating that many individuals underestimate their knowledge of Parkinson's. To increase the awareness of Parkinson's disease among young adults, educational programs and awareness campaigns should start up.

INTRODUCTION

Parkinson's disease is a debilitating neurological condition that is associated with tremors, muscular rigidity, sleep disturbances, speech changes, and other symptoms that can greatly diminish quality of life (1-8). Parkinson's disease still has no cure, but standard of care can be improved significantly through education of caregivers (9).

Numerous studies have been conducted to assess knowledge and awareness levels of young adults with regards to Parkinson's disease (10-14). These studies appear to demonstrate that young adults are relatively well-informed about the condition. Studies by Chow et al. in London, Canada (10) and Viehweger et al. in Waterloo, Canada (12) demonstrate that over half of young adults are knowledgeable about Parkinson's disease. This is reassuring, considering that a much smaller proportion of young adults actually have a family member suffering from the disease (10-14).

While young adults appear to be well-aware, it is interesting that awareness levels vary in different regions of Canada and the world. The purpose of this study is to assess the awareness levels of young adults in Kingston, Ontario, Canada.

OUR STUDY

A questionnaire was circulated to young adults in Kingston, Canada, through social media platforms. The first page of the survey contained the consent form which outlined that completing the forms was voluntary. The subsequent page inquired about demographic information. The final page evaluated the participant's actual and perceived awareness of Parkinson's disease (15).

Descriptive statistics were used to analyze participant demographics and the number of correct/incorrect answers. To determine whether there was a difference in categorical questions, Fisher exact tests were applied with respect to age groups (under and over 20 year olds), sexes (males and females), family history with the disease (affected and not affected by Parkinson's disease) and the frequency of visiting their family members (less than and over 10 visits a year). ANOVA procedures were used to evaluate the average number of correct answers between the subgroups. All analyses were conducted using the Statistical Analysis Software (SAS Version 9.4 for Windows) (15).

FINDINGS

The survey was consented and completed by a total of 24 people. 16 (67%) of respondents were between 18 and 19 years old, 6 (25%) were between 20 and 22 years old and the remaining 2 (8%) respondents were over 22 years old. 5 (21%) respondents were male and 19 (79%) were female. There were 5 (21%) participants who reported having a family member who was affected by Parkinson's disease, while 19 (79%) did not have an affected member. Of the 5 respondents with affected family members, 3 (60%) indicated that they visited the affected member over 20 times a year, while 1 (20%) respondent reported visiting less than 3 times a year and the final respondent (20%) stated that they visited between 3 and 10 times a year (see Table 1).

Only a third of respondents were confident about their knowledge of Parkinson's disease. 38% of participants correctly identified that the cause of Parkinson's disease is unknown, 88% stated that there is no cure to the disease and only treatment of symptoms and 38% commented that there is no specific test to diagnose Parkinson's disease. 83% said that stress can worsen the condition, 54% stated that exercise may slow the progression of Parkinson's disease, 92% correctly chose that Parkinson's does not only affect old people and 42% of respondents recognized that men and women are not equally as likely to be affected by Parkinson's disease. 54% stated that there is a correlation between Parkinson's and depression. Overall, 39% of respondents had adequate knowledge of the disease, and the average knowledge score was 4.88 out of 8 (see Table 2).

Table 1. Demographics

Demographic	**n = 24**
Age Group	
Under 18 years old	0 (0%)
18-19 years old	16 (67%)
20-22 years old	6 (25%)
Over 22 years old	2 (8%)
Sex	
Male	5 (21%)
Female	19 (79%)
Prefer not to say	0 (0%)
Family member affected by Parkinson's disease	
Yes	5 (21%)
No	19 (79%)
Number of visits to Parkinson's family member a year (n = 5)	
Less than 3	1 (20%)
3-10	1 (20%)
10-20	0 (0%)
20+	3 (60%)

Table 2. Perceived and actual knowledge

Question Item	**n = 24**
"I believe I am knowledgeable about Parkinson's disease"	
Agree	8 (33%)
Disagree	6 (25%)
Neutral	10 (42%)
"The cause of Parkinson's disease is unknown"	
True	9 (38%)
False	8 (33%)
Not Sure	7 (29%)
"There is no cure to the disease, only treatments of symptoms"	
True	21 (88%)
False	0 (0%)
Not Sure	3 (13%)
"There is no specific test to diagnose Parkinson's disease"	
True	9 (38%)
False	10 (42%)
Not Sure	5 (21%)
"Stress can worsen the condition"	
True	20 (83%)
False	0 (0%)
Not Sure	4 (17%)
"Exercise may slow the progression of Parkinson's disease"	
True	13 (54%)
False	3 (13%)
Not Sure	8 (33%)
"Parkinson's only affects old people"	
True	0 (0%)
False	22 (92%)
Not Sure	2 (8%)
"Men and women are equally as likely to be affected by Parkinson's"	
True	7 (29%)
False	10 (42%)
Not Sure	7 (29%)
"There is no correlation between Parkinson's and depression"	
True	2 (8%)
False	13 (54%)
Not Sure	9 (38%)

Table 2. (Continued)

Question Item	n = 24
Knowledge Score	
Not Knowledgeable (0-4)	10 (42%)
Satisfactory (5-6)	11 (26%)
Knowledgeable (7-8)	3 (13%)
Mean ± SD	4.88 ± 1.78

Subgroup analyses show that there are no statistically significant differences between the perceived and actual knowledge of respondents. 31% of respondents under 20 years old and 38% of those over the age of 20 believed they were knowledgeable about Parkinson's disease ($p = 0.7430$). 25% and 63% of those under 20 and over 20 respectively reported that the cause of Parkinson's disease is unknown ($p = 0.2661$). 88% of both groups commented that there is no cure to the disease, only treatment of symptoms ($p = 0.9999$). 31% of those under 20 and 50% of those above 20 identified that there is no specific test to diagnose Parkinson's disease ($p = 0.7430$). 81% and 88% of those under 20 and over 20 respectively remarked that stress can worsen the condition ($p = 0.9999$). 44% of those under 20 and 75% of those above 20 stated that exercise may slow the progression of Parkinson's disease ($p = 0.3603$), and 88% of those under 20 and all participants above 20 reported that Parkinson's does not only affect old people ($p = 0.5362$). 44% and 38% of those under and over 20 respectively said men and women were not equally likely to be affected by the disease ($p = 0.8741$). 56% and 50% of those above and below 20 respectively said there is a correlation between Parkinson's and depression ($p = 0.5637$). Overall, 56% of those under 20 and 63% of those above 20 had a sufficient level of knowledge regarding the disease ($p = 0.5181$). The mean score for those below 20 was 4.56 and the mean for those above 20 was 5.50 ($p = 0.2301$) (see Table 3).

Table 3. Perceived and actual knowledge - by subgroups

Question Item	Under 20 n = 16	Over 20 n = 8	p-value
"I believe I am knowledgeable about Parkinson's disease"			0.7430
Agree	5 (31%)	3 (38%)	
Disagree	5 (31%)	1 (13%)	
Neutral	6 (38%)	4 (50%)	
"The cause of Parkinson's disease is unknown"			0.2661
True	4 (25%)	5 (63%)	
False	6 (38%)	2 (25%)	
Not Sure	6 (38%)	1 (13%)	
"There is no cure to the disease, only treatments of symptoms"			0.9999
True	14 (88%)	7 (88%)	
False	0 (0%)	0 (0%)	
Not Sure	2 (13%)	1 (13%)	
"There is no specific test to diagnose Parkinson's disease"			0.7430
True	5 (31%)	4 (50%)	
False	7 (44%)	3 (38%)	
Not Sure	4 (25%)	1 (13%)	
"Stress can worsen the condition"			0.9999
True	13 (81%)	7 (88%)	
False	0 (0%)	0 (0%)	
Not Sure	3 (19%)	1 (13%)	
"Exercise may slow the progression of Parkinson's disease"			0.3603
True	7 (44%)	6 (75%)	
False	3 (19%)	0 (0%)	
Not Sure	6 (38%)	2 (25%)	
"Parkinson's only affects old people"			0.5362
True	0 (0%)	0 (0%)	
False	14 (88%)	8 (100%)	
Not Sure	2 (13%)	0 (0%)	
"Men and women are equally as likely to be affected by Parkinson's"			0.8741
True	4 (25%)	3 (38%)	
False	7 (44%)	3 (38%)	
Not Sure	5 (31%)	2 (25%)	

Table 3. (Continued)

Question Item	**Under 20** **n = 16**	**Over 20** **n = 8**	**p-value**
"There is no correlation between Parkinson's and depression"			0.5637
True	2 (13%)	0 (0%)	
False	9 (56%)	4 (50%)	
Not Sure	5 (31%)	4 (50%)	
Knowledge Score			
Not Knowledgeable (0-4)	7 (44%)	3 (38%)	0.5181
Satisfactory (5-6)	8 (50%)	3 (38%)	
Knowledgeable (7-8)	1 (6%)	2 (25%)	
Mean ± SD	4.56 ± 1.79	5.50 ± 1.69	0.2301
Question Item	**Males** **n = 5**	**Females** **n = 19**	
"I believe I am knowledgeable about Parkinson's disease"			0.2010
Agree	1 (20%)	7 (37%)	
Disagree	0 (0%)	6 (32%)	
Neutral	4 (80%)	6 (32%)	
"The cause of Parkinson's disease is unknown"			0.4565
True	1 (20%)	8 (42%)	
False	3 (60%)	5 (26%)	
Not Sure	1 (20%)	6 (32%)	
"There is no cure to the disease, only treatments of symptoms"			0.9999
True	5 (100%)	16 (84%)	
False	0 (0%)	0 (0%)	
Not Sure	0 (0%)	3 (16%)	
"There is no specific test to diagnose Parkinson's disease"			0.6824
True	2 (40%)	7 (37%)	
False	3 (60%)	7 (37%)	
Not Sure	0 (0%)	5 (26%)	
"Stress can worsen the condition"			0.9999
True	4 (80%)	16 (84%)	
False	0 (0%)	0 (0%)	
Not Sure	1 (20%)	3 (16%)	

Question Item	Males n = 5	Females n = 19	
"Exercise may slow the progression of Parkinson's disease"			0.6036
True	4 (80%)	9 (47%)	
False	0 (0%)	2 (11%)	
Not Sure	1 (20%)	8 (42%)	
"Parkinson's only affects old people"			0.9999
True	0 (0%)	0 (0%)	
False	5 (100%)	17 (89%)	
Not Sure	0 (0%)	2 (11%)	
"Men and women are equally as likely to be affected by Parkinson's"			0.0125
True	4 (80%)	3 (16%)	
False	0 (0%)	10 (53%)	
Not Sure	1 (20%)	6 (32%)	
"There is no correlation between Parkinson's and depression"			0.7671
True	0 (0%)	2 (11%)	
False	2 (40%)	10 (53%)	
Not Sure	3 (60%)	7 (37%)	
Knowledge Score			
Not Knowledgeable (0-4)	3 (60%)	7 (37%)	0.6506
Satisfactory (5-6)	2 (40%)	9 (47%)	
Knowledgeable (7-8)	0 (0%)	3 (16%)	
Mean ± SD	4.80 ± 1.10	4.89 ± 1.94	0.9224
Question Item	**Affected n = 5**	**Unaffected n = 19**	
"I believe I am knowledgeable about Parkinson's disease"			0.2010
Agree	1 (20%)	7 (37%)	
Disagree	4 (80%)	6 (32%)	
Neutral	0 (0%)	6 (32%)	
"The cause of Parkinson's disease is unknown"			0.3142
True	3 (60%)	6 (32%)	
False	2 (40%)	6 (32%)	
Not Sure	0 (0%)	7 (37%)	

Table 3. (Continued)

Question Item	Affected n = 5	Unaffected n = 19	
"There is no cure to the disease, only treatments of symptoms"			0.9999
True	5 (100%)	16 (84%)	
False	0 (0%)	0 (0%)	
Not Sure	0 (0%)	3 (16%)	
"There is no specific test to diagnose Parkinson's disease"			0.9999
True	2 (40%)	7 (37%)	
False	2 (40%)	8 (42%)	
Not Sure	1 (20%)	4 (21%)	
"Stress can worsen the condition"			0.2933
True	4 (80%)	16 (84%)	
False	1 (20%)	0 (0%)	
Not Sure	0 (0%)	3 (16%)	
"Exercise may slow the progression of Parkinson's disease"			0.8116
True	3 (60%)	10 (53%)	
False	1 (20%)	2 (11%)	
Not Sure	1 (20%)	7 (37%)	
"Parkinson's only affects old people"			0.9999
True	0 (0%)	0 (0%)	
False	5 (100%)	17 (89%)	
Not Sure	0 (0%)	2 (11%)	
"Men and women are equally as likely to be affected by Parkinson's"			0.9999
True	2 (40%)	5 (26%)	
False	2 (40%)	8 (42%)	
Not Sure	1 (20%)	6 (32%)	
"There is no correlation between Parkinson's and depression"			0.6036
True	0 (0%)	2 (11%)	
False	4 (80%)	9 (47%)	
Not Sure	1 (20%)	8 (42%)	
Knowledge Score			
Not Knowledgeable (0-4)	2 (40%)	8 (42%)	0.9999
Satisfactory (5-6)	2 (40%)	9 (47%)	
Knowledgeable (7-8)	1 (20%)	2 (11%)	
Mean ± SD	5.60 ± 1.67	4.68 ± 1.80	0.3142

Question Item	**Less than 10 visits n = 2**	**More than 10 visits n = 3**	
"I believe I am knowledgeable about Parkinson's disease"			0.9999
Agree	0 (0%)	1 (33%)	
Disagree	0 (0%)	0 (0%)	
Neutral	2 (100%)	2 (67%)	
"The cause of Parkinson's disease is unknown"			0.9999
True	1 (50%)	2 (67%)	
False	1 (50%)	1 (33%)	
Not Sure	0 (0%)	0 (0%)	
"There is no cure to the disease, only treatments of symptoms"			0.9999
True	2 (100%)	3 (100%)	
False	0 (0%)	0 (0%)	
Not Sure	0 (0%)	0 (0%)	
"There is no specific test to diagnose Parkinson's disease"			0.9999
True	1 (50%)	1 (33%)	
False	1 (50%)	1 (33%)	
Not Sure	0 (0%)	1 (33%)	
"Stress can worsen the condition"			0.9999
True	2 (100%)	2 (67%)	
False	0 (0%)	0 (0%)	
Not Sure	0 (0%)	1 (33%)	
"Exercise may slow the progression of Parkinson's disease"			0.9999
True	1 (50%)	2 (67%)	
False	1 (50%)	0 (0%)	
Not Sure	0 (0%)	1 (33%)	
"Parkinson's only affects old people"			0.9999
True	0 (0%)	0 (0%)	
False	2 (100%)	3 (100%)	
Not Sure	0 (0%)	0 (0%)	
"Men and women are equally as likely to be affected by Parkinson's"			0.9999
True	1 (50%)	1 (33%)	
False	1 (50%)	1 (33%)	
Not Sure	0 (0%)	1 (33%)	

Table 3. (Continued)

Question Item	Less than 10 visits n = 2	More than 10 visits n = 3	
"There is no correlation between Parkinson's and depression"			0.9999
True	0 (0%)	0 (0%)	
False	2 (100%)	2 (67%)	
Not Sure	0 (0%)	1 (33%)	
Knowledge Score			
Not Knowledgeable (0-4)	0 (0%)	2 (67%)	0.2000
Satisfactory (5-6)	2 (100%)	0 (0%)	
Knowledgeable (7-8)	0 (0%)	1 (33%)	
Mean ± SD	6.00 ± 0.00	5.33 ± 2.31	0.7232

There was also no major difference in knowledge between males and females. The only statistically significant component was that females were more likely to identify that men and women are not equally as likely to be affected by the disease; 0% of males and 53% of females reported this ($p = 0.0125$). 37% of females and 20% of males believed they were knowledgeable about Parkinson's disease ($p = 0.2010$). 20% and 42% of males and females respectively identified that the cause of Parkinson's disease is unknown ($p = 0.4565$). 100% and 84% said there is no cure to the disease ($p = 0.9999$), 40% and 37% commented that there is no specific test to diagnose the disease ($p = 0.6824$), 80% and 84% reported that stress can worsen the condition ($p = 0.9999$), 80% and 47% reported that exercise may slow the progression of the disease ($p = 0.6036$), 100% and 89% stated that Parkinson's does not only affect old people ($p = 0.9999$) and 40% and 53% said there is a correlation between Parkinson's and depression ($p = 0.7671$). Overall, 40% and 63% of males and females respectively had an adequate knowledge of the disease ($p = 0.6506$), while the mean scores were 4.80 for males and 4.89 for females (p = 0.9224) (see Table 3).

There is also no difference in knowledge between those with an affected family member and those without one. 20% of those with an affected member believed they were knowledgeable while 37% of those without one believed they were knowledgeable (p = 0.2010). 60% and 32% of those with an affected member and those without an affected member respectively said the cause of Parkinson's disease is unknown (p = 0.3142). 100% and 84% of the same groups commented that there is no cure for the disease (p = 0.9999). 40% and 37% said there is no specific test to diagnose for Parkinson's (p = 0.9999), 80% and 84% remarked that stress can worsen the condition (p = 0.2933), 60% and 53% said exercise may slow the progression of the disease (p = 0.8116) and 100% and 89% reported that Parkinson's does not only affects old people (p = 0.9999). 40% and 42% correctly identified that men and women are not equally as likely to be affected by the disease (p = 0.9999) and 80% and 47% reported that there exists a correlation between Parkinson's disease and depression (p = 0.6036). Overall, 60% and 58% of those with an affected family member and those without one had an acceptable level of knowledge about the disease (p = 0.9999). The mean score for those with an affected member was 5.60 while the mean for those without an affected member was 4.68 (p = 0.3142) (see Table 3).

Again, there is no difference among those with an affected family member between those who visited less than 10 times per year and those who visited more than 10 times a year. 0% of those with less than 10 visits and 33% of those with more than 10 visits thought they were knowledgeable about the disease (p = 0.9999). 50% of those who visited less than 10 times and 67% of those who visited more than 10 times said the cause of Parkinson's disease is unknown (p = 0.9999). 100% of both groups reported that there is no cure to the disease (p = 0.9999). Half of those with less than ten visits and a third of those with more than ten visits said there is no specific tests to diagnose the disease (p = 0.9999). 100% and 67% reported that stress can worsen the condition (p-0.9999), 50% and 66% said exercise may slow the progression of the disease (p = 0.9999), 100% of both groups reported that Parkinson's does not only affect old people (0.9999), 50% and 33% said that men and women are not equally as likely to be affected by the disease (p = 0.9999), and 100% and 67% commented that there is a correlation between Parkinson's and depression (p = 0.9999). All of those who visited less than 10 times and 33% of those who visited more than 10 times had an adequate knowledge of the disease (p = 0.2000). The mean score for those with less than 10 visits was 6 and the mean for those with more than 10 visits is 5.33 (p = 0.7232) (see Table 3).

DISCUSSION

39% of respondents were knowledgeable about the disease; this is greater than the 33% who believed they were knowledgeable and the 21% who had a family member affected by Parkinson's disease. The calculated knowledge scores are in line with previously reported trends, thus validating that young adults are sufficiently aware of the disease. Despite this, there is much room to increase awareness among this population which will result in better care in the future.

There is no difference in awareness between the subgroups. This study confirms the previously noted trends, which report that awareness between younger and older individuals, males and females and affected and unaffected are equal.

This study is not without limitations - since it is a survey study, there is a possibility of response and sampling bias. Additionally, the small sample size resulted in some analyses with reduced statistical power (i.e., less than 10 visits and more than 10 visits).

In conclusion, 39% possess an adequate knowledge of the disease, which is greater than the 33% who believed they were knowledgeable and the 21% who had a family member affected by the disease. Implementing educational programs and campaigns will greatly benefit this population as they will be able to better care for the elderly in the future.

REFERENCES

[1] Polymeropoulos MH, Lavedan C, Leroy E, Ide SE, Dehejia A, Dutra A, et al. Mutation in the α-synuclein gene identified in families with Parkinson's disease. Science 1997;276:2045-7.

[2] Global Parkinson's Disease Survey Steering Committee. Factors impacting on quality of life in Parkinson's disease: results from an international survey. Mov Disord 2002;17:60-7.

[3] Chaudhuri KR, Schapira AHV, Martinez-Martin P. The holistic management of Parkinson's using a novel non-motor symptom scale and questionnaire. Adv Clin Neurosci Rehabil 2004;4:20-4.

[4] Aarsland D, Larsen JP, Tandberg E, Laake K. Predictors of nursing home placement in Parkinson's disease: a population-based, prospective study. J Am Geriatr Soc 2000;48:938-42.

[5] Witjas T, Kaphan E, Azulay JP, Blin O, Ceccaldi M, Pouget J, et al. Nonmotor fluctuations in Parkinson's disease: frequent and disabling. Neurology 2002;59(3):408-13.

[6] Schrag A, Jahanshahi N, Quinn N. What contributes to quality of life in patients with Parkinson's disease? J Neurol Neurosurg Psychiatry 2000;69:308-12.

[7] Findley L, Aujla M, Bain PG, Baker M, Beech C, Bowman C, et al. Direct economic impact of Parkinson's disease: a research survey in the United Kingdom. Mov Disord 2003;18(10):1139-45.

[8] Hagell P, Nordling S, Reimer J, Grabowski M, Persson U. Resource use and costs in a Swedish cohort of patients with Parkinson's disease. Mov Disord 2002;17:1213-20.

[9] Chow R, Borean M, Hollenberg D, Merrick J. How aware/knowledgeable are young adults about Parkinson's disease? J Pain Manage 2019;12(1), in press.

[10] Chow R, Viehweger J, Trasente V, Borean M, Hollenberg D, Lam M, et al. Awareness of Parkinson's disease among young adults in London, Canada. J Pain Manage 2019;12(1), in press.

[11] Ho S, Viehweger J, Trasente V, Ho C, Ng W, Wong M, et al. Awareness of Parkinson's disease among young adults in Toronto, Canada. J Pain Manage 2019;12(1), in press.

[12] Viehweger J, Chow R, Trasente V, Duarte N, Borean M, Hollenberg D, et al. Awareness of Parkinson's disease among young adults in Waterloo, Canada. J Pain Manage 2019;12(1), in press.
[13] Ho S, Viehweger J, Trasente V, Borean M, Hollenberg D, Ferguson T, et al. Awareness of Parkinson's disease among young adults in Halifax, Canada. J Pain Manage 2019;12(1), in press.
[14] Anpalagan T, Chow R, Viehweger J, Trasente V, Borean M, Hollenberg D, et al. Awareness of Parkinson's disease among young adults in Asia. J Pain Manage 2019;12(1), in press.
[15] Chow R, Borean M, Hollenberg D. Awareness of Parkinson's disease: About the survey instrument. J Pain Manage 2019;12(1), in press.

Section two: United States, Ireland and Asia

In: Parkinson's Disease
Editors: Ronald Chow, et al.
ISBN: 978-1-53612-745-4

Chapter 8

AWARENESS OF PARKINSON'S DISEASE AMONG YOUNG ADULTS IN NEW YORK STATE, UNITED STATES

Jaclyn Viehweger, BMSc(C), Victoria Trasente, BA(C), Neal Ganguli, BSc(C), Ray Kang, BSc(C), Michael Borean, BMSc(C), Drew Hollenberg, BMSc(C), Tharani Anpalagan, BMSc(C), Anna Rzepka, BMSc(C) and Ronald Chow*, BMSc(C)
Infinitas Research Group, London, Ontario, Canada

The aim of our study was to further add to the literature about this topic by studying young adults in New York State, USA. A questionnaire was circulated via social media outlets to young adults in New York State, USA. The survey was voluntary and the consent form on the first page acknowledged that there are no benefits/costs to participants. The second page collected demographic information and the third page was used to determine the actual and perceived awareness of Parkinson's disease. A

* Correspondence: Ronald Chow BMSc(C), Infinitas Research Group, London, Ontario, Canada. Email: rchow48@uwo.ca.

total of 13 people consented and completed the study. 46% were knowledgeable about the disease, which is greater than the 15% who believed they were knowledgeable and the 8% who have a family member affected by the disease. Interpreting the knowledge level in lieu of the other statistics confirms the trend that young adults seem to be adequately aware of the disease. The statistics suggest that there is still plenty of room to improve awareness, and educational programs should be designed to increase the awareness of young adults so they can better care the disease.

INTRODUCTION

Parkinson's disease is an incurable disease, at the moment, with the best treatments only alleviating symptom burden. The other best method to improve quality of life of these patients is to understand their disease and disease progression, and to provide individualized care (1).

Studies have been conducted to look into the awareness level of young adults - this population should be able to assist affected individuals at the present time and will also be more heavily relied upon in the future to support those who are affected by the disease (1).

A study by Chow et al. (2) looked at young adults in London, Canada, and reported that they were adequately aware of the disease. While 27% had family members affected by the disease, a higher 41% of respondents believed they were knowledgeable and an even higher 54% were deemed knowledgeable about the disease (2). Similar findings were reported among young adults in Toronto (Canada), Waterloo (Canada), Halifax (Canada) and Asia (3-6), where there seems to exist a trend that young adults are adequately aware about the disease.

The studies do show that there exists variation by geographic location within Canada and between Canada and Asia, with each area boasting a difference awareness level and different percentage of the population with relatives affected by the disease. The aim of our study was to further add to the literature about this topic by studying young adults in New York State, USA.

OUR QUESTIONNAIRE

A questionnaire was circulated via social media outlets to young adults in New York State, USA. The survey was voluntary and the consent form on the first page acknowledged that there are no benefits/costs to participants. The second page collected demographic information and the third page was used to determine the actual and perceived awareness of Parkinson's disease (7).

Descriptive statistics were used to disclose participant demographics, and the number of correct/incorrect answers. Fisher exact tests were used to determine whether there was a difference in categorical questions between age groups (under and over 20 years old), gender groups (males and females), familial ties (affected and not affected by Parkinson's disease) and the frequency of visiting their family members (less than and over 10 visits a year). ANOVA procedures compared the average number of correct answers between the subgroups. All analyses were conducted using the Statistical Analysis Software (SAS Version 9.4 for Windows) (7).

FINDINGS

A total of 13 people consented and completed the study. 4 (31%) were between 20 and 22 years old, and the remaining 9 were split evenly across the other three cohorts of under 18 years old (23%), 18-19 years old (23%) and over 22 years old (23%). 23% identified as male, 69% reported they were female, and 8% did not disclose their sex. 8% had a family member affected by the disease, and visited that family member more than 20 times a year (see Table 1).

Table 1. Demographics

Demographic	n = 13
Age Group	
Under 18 years old	3 (23%)
18-19 years old	3 (23%)
20-22 years old	4 (31%)
Over 22 years old	3 (23%)
Sex	
Male	3 (23%)
Female	9 (69%)
Prefer not to say	1 (8%)
Family member affected by Parkinson's disease	
Yes	1 (8%)
No	12 (92%)
Number of visits to Parkinson's family member a year (n = 1)	
Less than 3	0 (0%)
3-10	0 (0%)
10-20	0 (0%)
20+	1 (100%)

Table 2. Perceived and actual knowledge

Question Item	n = 13
"I believe I am knowledgeable about Parkinson's disease"	
Agree	2 (15%)
Disagree	5 (38%)
Neutral	6 (46%)
"The cause of Parkinson's disease is unknown"	
True	5 (38%)
False	2 (15%)
Not Sure	6 (46%)
"There is no cure to the disease, only treatments of symptoms"	
True	9 (69%)
False	1 (8%)
Not Sure	3 (23%)
"There is no specific test to diagnose Parkinson's disease"	
True	3 (23%)
False	3 (23%)
Not Sure	7 (54%)

Question Item	**n = 13**
"Stress can worsen the condition"	
True	8 (62%)
False	1 (8%)
Not Sure	4 (31%)
"Exercise may slow the progression of Parkinson's disease"	
True	7 (54%)
False	0 (0%)
Not Sure	6 (46%)
"Parkinson's only affects old people"	
True	1 (8%)
False	11 (85%)
Not Sure	1 (8%)
"Men and women are equally as likely to be affected by	
Parkinson's"	3 (23%)
True	3 (23%)
False	7 (54%)
Not Sure	
"There is no correlation between Parkinson's and depression"	
True	2 (15%)
False	6 (46%)
Not Sure	5 (38%)
Knowledge Score	
Not Knowledgeable (0-4)	7 (54%)
Satisfactory (5-6)	4 (31%)
Knowledgeable (7-8)	2 (15%)
Mean ± SD	4.00 ± 2.20

Only 15% believed they were knowledgeable about the disease. 38% correctly noted that the cause is unknown, 69% responded that there is no cure to the disease, 23% concluded that there is no specific diagnostic test, 62% indicated that stress can worsen the condition, and 54% answered that exercise may slow the progression of the disease. 85% noted that it does not only affect old people, 23% identified that men and women are not equally as likely to be affected by the disease and 46% noted there is a correlation between the disease and depression. Overall, 46% were aware of the disease, with the average score being 4.00 out of 8 (see Table 2).

Subgroup analysis by age revealed no difference in perceived and actual awareness. 17% and 14% of those under 20 and over 20, respectively, indicated that they believe they are aware of the disease ($p = 0.9999$). 33% and 43% of the same groups, respectively, noted that the cause is unknown ($p = 0.5105$), 67% and 57% indicated that there is no cure to the disease ($p = 0.9999$), 17% and 29% responded that there is no diagnostic test ($p = 0.9999$), 67% and 43% concluded that stress can worsen the condition ($p = 0.5921$), and 67% and 43% noted that exercise may slow the progression of the disease ($p = 0.5921$). 83% and 86% responded in the negative to indicate that Parkinson's does not only affect old people ($p = 0.9999$), while 17% and 29% noted that men and women are not equally as likely to be affected by the disease ($p = 0.9999$) and 50% and 43% noted that there does exist a correlation between the disease and depression ($p = 0.9999$). Overall, 50% and 57% were not knowledgeable ($p = 0.3718$), and they had average scores of 4.17 and 3.86, respectively ($p = 0.8121$) (see Table 3).

Males and females seemed to be equally aware of the disease. 0% and 11% of males and females, respectively, believed they were knowledgeable ($p = 0.6591$). 0% and 44% answered that the cause is unknown ($p = 0.3455$), 33% and 78% noted that there is no cure to the disease ($p = 0.2364$), 33% and 11% concluded that there is no specific test to diagnose Parkinson's disease ($p = 0.7136$), and 33% and 67% reported that stress can worsen the condition ($p = 0.6182$). The fact that exercise may slow the progression of the disease was identified by 33% and 56% ($p = 0.9999$), while 67% and 100% indicated that it does not only affect old people ($p = 0.2500$), 33% and 22% noted that men and women are not equally as likely to be affected by the disease ($p = 0.9999$) and 67% and 44% noted that there is a correlation between the disease and depression ($p = 0.9999$). 67% and 56% were not knowledgeable ($p = 0.7136$); average scores for males and females were 3.00 and 4.22, respectively ($p = 0.4482$) (see Table 3).

Table 3. Perceived and actual knowledge - by subgroups

Question Item	Under 20 n = 6	Over 20 n = 7	p-value
"I believe I am knowledgeable about Parkinson's disease"			0.9999
Agree	1 (17%)	1 (14%)	
Disagree	4 (67%)	5 (71%)	
Neutral	1 (17%)	1 (14%)	
"The cause of Parkinson's disease is unknown"			0.5105
True	2 (33%)	3 (43%)	
False	3 (50%)	1 (14%)	
Not Sure	1 (17%)	3 (43%)	
"There is no cure to the disease, only treatments of symptoms"			0.9999
True	4 (67%)	4 (57%)	
False	0 (0%)	1 (14%)	
Not Sure	2 (33%)	2 (29%)	
"There is no specific test to diagnose Parkinson's disease"			0.9999
True	1 (17%)	2 (29%)	
False	2 (33%)	1 (17%)	
Not Sure	3 (50%)	4 (57%)	
"Stress can worsen the condition"			0.5921
True	4 (67%)	3 (43%)	
False	0 (0%)	2 (29%)	
Not Sure	2 (33%)	2 (29%)	
"Exercise may slow the progression of Parkinson's disease"			0.5921
True	4 (67%)	3 (43%)	
False	0 (0%)	0 (0%)	
Not Sure	2 (33%)	4 (57%)	
"Parkinson's only affects old people"			0.9999
True	1 (17%)	0 (0%)	
False	5 (83%)	6 (86%)	
Not Sure	0 (0%)	1 (17%)	
"Men and women are equally as likely to be affected by Parkinson's"			0.9999
True	2 (33%)	1 (17%)	
False	1 (17%)	2 (29%)	
Not Sure	3 (50%)	4 (57%)	

Table 3. (Continued)

Question Item	**Under 20** **n = 6**	**Over 20** **n = 7**	**p-value**
"There is no correlation between Parkinson's and depression"			0.9999
True	1 (17%)	1 (17%)	
False	3 (50%)	3 (43%)	
Not Sure	2 (33%)	3 (43%)	
Knowledge Score			0.3718
Not Knowledgeable (0-4)	3 (50%)	4 (57%)	
Satisfactory (5-6)	3 (50%)	1 (17%)	
Knowledgeable (7-8)	0 (0%)	2 (29%)	
Mean ± SD	4.17 ± 1.83	3.86 ± 2.61	0.8121
Question Item	**Males** **n = 3**	**Females** **n = 9**	
"I believe I am knowledgeable about Parkinson's disease"			0.6591
Agree	0 (0%)	1 (11%)	
Disagree	2 (67%)	3 (33%)	
Neutral	1 (33%)	5 (56%)	
"The cause of Parkinson's disease is unknown"			0.3455
True	0 (0%)	4 (44%)	
False	1 (33%)	1 (11%)	
Not Sure	2 (67%)	4 (44%)	
"There is no cure to the disease, only treatments of symptoms"			0.2364
True	1 (33%)	7 (78%)	
False	0 (0%)	1 (11%)	
Not Sure	2 (67%)	1 (11%)	
"There is no specific test to diagnose Parkinson's disease"			0.7136
True	1 (33%)	1 (11%)	
False	0 (0%)	3 (33%)	
Not Sure	2 (67%)	5 (56%)	
"Stress can worsen the condition"			0.6182
True	1 (33%)	6 (67%)	
False	0 (0%)	1 (11%)	
Not Sure	2 (67%)	2 (22%)	

Question Item	**Males** **n = 3**	**Females** **n = 9**	
"Exercise may slow the progression of Parkinson's disease"			0.9999
True	1 (33%)	5 (56%)	
False	0 (0%)	0 (0%)	
Not Sure	2 (67%)	4 (44%)	
"Parkinson's only affects old people"			0.2500
True	0 (0%)	0 (0%)	
False	2 (67%)	9 (100%)	
Not Sure	1 (33%)	0 (0%)	
"Men and women are equally as likely to be affected by Parkinson's"			0.9999
True	0 (0%)	2 (22%)	
False	1 (33%)	2 (22%)	
Not Sure	2 (67%)	5 (56%)	
"There is no correlation between Parkinson's and depression"			0.9999
True	0 (0%)	1 (11%)	
False	2 (67%)	4 (44%)	
Not Sure	1 (33%)	4 (44%)	
Knowledge Score			0.7136
Not Knowledgeable (0-4)	2 (67%)	5 (56%)	
Satisfactory (5-6)	0 (0%)	3 (33%)	
Knowledgeable (7-8)	1 (33%)	1 (11%)	
Mean ± SD	3.00 ± 3.61	4.22 ± 1.86	0.4482

DISCUSSION

46% were knowledgeable about the disease, which is greater than the 15% who believed they were knowledgeable and the 8% who have a family member affected by the disease. Interpreting the knowledge level in lieu of the other statistics confirms the trend that young adults seem to be adequately aware of the disease. The statistics suggest that there is still plenty of room to improve awareness, and educational programs should be designed to increase the awareness of young adults so they can better care the disease.

There fails to exist a difference in awareness by subgroup analyses. Our study was not able to look into whether those with a family member affected by the disease were more aware as others have in the past (2-4), but our study did validate that awareness between younger and older individuals, and also males and females, are equivalent.

This study was not without limitations. As this is a survey study, there exists the possibility of a response and sampling bias. Additionally, due to the small sample size, certain statistical analyses were not conducted (i.e., subgroup analyses between those affected and not affected by the disease) and other analyses had reduced statistical power (i.e., males vs females).

In conclusion, 46% were knowledgeable about the disease, which is greater than the 15% who believed they were knowledgeable and the 8% who have a family member affected by the disease. Educational programs should be designed to increase the awareness of young adults so they can better care the disease.

References

[1] Chow R, Borean M, Hollenberg D, Merrick J. How aware/knowledgeable are young adults about Parkinson's disease? J Pain Manage 2019;12(1), in press.

[2] Chow R, Viehweger J, Trasente V, Borean M, Hollenberg D, Lam M, et al. Awareness of Parkinson's disease among young adults in London, Canada. J Pain Manage 2019;12(1), in press.

[3] Ho S, Viehweger J, Trasente V, Ho C, Ng W, Wong M, et al. Awareness of Parkinson's disease among young adults in Toronto, Canada. J Pain Manage 2019;12(1), in press.

[4] Viehweger J, Chow R, Trasente V, Duarte N, Borean M, Hollenberg D, et al. Awareness of Parkinson's disease among young adults in Waterloo, Canada. J Pain Manage 2019;12(1), in press.

[5] Ho S, Viehweger J, Trasente V, Borean M, Hollenberg D, Ferguson T, et al. Awareness of Parkinson's disease among young adults in Halifax, Canada. J Pain Manage 2019;12(1), in press.

[6] Anpalagan T, Chow R, Viehweger J, Trasente V, Borean M, Hollenberg D, et al. Awareness of Parkinson's disease among young adults in Asia. J Pain Manage 2019;12(1), in press.

[7] Chow R, Borean M, Hollenberg D. Awareness of Parkinson's disease: About the survey instrument. J Pain Manage 2019;12(1), in press.

In: Parkinson's Disease
Editors: Ronald Chow, et al.
ISBN: 978-1-53612-745-4

Chapter 9

Awareness of Parkinson's Disease among Young Adults in Dublin, Ireland

Drew Hollenberg, BMSc(C),
Jaclyn Viehweger, BMSc(C), Ronald Chow*, BMSc(C),
Anna Rzepka, BMSc(C), Victoria Trasente, BA(C),
Samuel Goh, MBChB(C), Michael Borean, BMSc(C)
and Tharani Anpalagan, BMSc(C)
Infinitas Research Group, London, Ontario, Canada

In this chapter we look into the awareness of young adults in Dublin, Ireland. A survey was circulated via social media outlets to young adults in Dublin, Ireland. Fisher exact tests were used to determine whether there was a difference in categorical questions between age groups (under and over 20 years old) and gender groups (males and females). ANOVA procedures compared the average number of correct answers between the

* Correspondence: Ronald Chow BMSc(C), Infinitas Research Group, London, Ontario, Canada. Email: rchow48@uwo.ca.

subgroups. A total of 15 young adults consented and completed the study. 53% were knowledgeable about the disease, much greater than the 27% who believed they were knowledgeable and also the 7% who had a family member affected by the disease. Educational programs should be setup to increase the awareness of the disease, as there is still room for improvement.

INTRODUCTION

Parkinson's disease was first described in detail in 1817 by James Parkinson (1). Since then, mankind has been able to better understand the neurodegenerative disease and the accompanying symptoms - tremors, muscular rigidity, bradykinesia, depression, psychosis, falls and sleep disturbances (2-10).

Even given greater understanding of the disease, there is yet to exist a cure to the debilitating disease. One of the best alternatives to improve standard of care is to educate and improve the awareness of the disease amongst caregivers, so they can provide more holistic care for the affected patients (11).

Many studies have looked into the awareness of young adults with respect to Parkinson's disease. The first study by Chow et al. (12) noted that young adults were adequately aware - a greater proportion of individuals are aware of the disease than the proportion of people who have family members affected by the disease (12). Follow-up studies in other geographic locations outside of London, Canada, suggested a similar trend but noticed variation in the reported portions (13-17).

There is yet to be a study that looks at the awareness of young adults in a European nation. The aim of this study was to look into the awareness of young adults in Dublin, Ireland.

OUR SURVEY

A survey was circulated via social media outlets to young adults in Dublin, Ireland. The survey was voluntary and the consent form on the first page acknowledged that there are no benefits/costs to participants. The second page collected demographic information and the third page was used to determine the actual and perceived awareness of Parkinson's disease (18).

Descriptive statistics were used to disclose participant demographics, and the number of correct/incorrect answers. Fisher exact tests were used to determine whether there was a difference in categorical questions between age groups (under and over 20 years old) and gender groups (males and females). ANOVA procedures compared the average number of correct answers between the subgroups. All analyses were conducted using the Statistical Analysis Software (SAS Version 9.4 for Windows) (18).

Table 1. Demographics

Demographic	**n = 15**
Age Group	
Under 18 years old	1 (7%)
18-19 years old	8 (53%)
20-22 years old	5 (33%)
Over 22 years old	1 (7%)
Sex	
Male	9 (60%)
Female	6 (40%)
Prefer not to say	0 (0%)
Family member affected by Parkinson's disease	
Yes	1 (7%)
No	14 (93%)
Number of visits to Parkinson's family member a year (n = 1)	
Less than 3	1 (100%)
3-10	0 (0%)
10-20	0 (0%)
20+	0 (0%)

FINDINGS

A total of 15 young adults consented and completed the study. 8 (53%) individuals noted they were between 18 and 19 years old, while 5 (33%) reported they were between 20 and 22 years old, 1 (7%) claimed they were under 18 years old, and another one (7%) claimed they were over 22 years old. Three-fifths were male, and two-fifths were female. Only one person (7%) had a family member affected by Parkinson's disease, and visited the family member less than 3 times a year (see Table 1).

27% believed they were knowledgeable about the disease. 47% correctly answered that the cause of the disease is unknown, 73% indicated that there is no cure to the disease, 27% noted that there is no specific diagnostic test, 60% concluded that stress can worsen the condition, and 60% proclaimed that exercise may slow the progression. 87% of young adults noted that Parkinson's does not only affect old people, 33% noted that the two sexes are not equally as likely to be affected, and 60% noted there is a correlation between the disease and depression. 20% were considered knowledgeable and 33% had satisfactory knowledge; the average score was 4.47 out of 8 (see Table 2).

Subgroup analyses by age revealed that age is not a predictor of perceived and actual knowledge level. 33% and 17% of those under and over 20 years old, respectively, believed they were knowledgeable ($p = 0.8127$). 44% and 50% noted that the cause of the disease is unknown ($p = 0.5717$), 89% and 50% concluded that there are only treatments of symptoms ($p = 0.1181$), 22% and 33% reported that there is no diagnostic test ($p = 0.9999$), 67% of both groups indicated that stress can worsen the condition ($p = 0.5220$), and 78% and 50% reported that exercise may slow the progression of the disease ($p = 0.2335$). 89% and 83% answered that the disease does not only affect old people ($p = 0.9999$), 22% and 50% noted that the sexes are not equally affected by the disease (p = 0.7483) and 78% and 33% concluded that there is a correlation between the disease and depression (p = 0.1357). 44% and 50% of the two groups were not knowledgeable (p = 0.5385); the mean scores were 4.67 and 4.17 (p = 0.6869) (see Table 3).

Males and females were equally knowledgeable about the disease. 33% of both groups, respectively, believed that they were not knowledgeable about the disease (p = 0.9999). 17% and 67% answered that there is no known cause (p = 0.1678), 67% and 78% concluded that there is no cure, 50% and 11% noted that there is no specific diagnostic test (p = 0.3487) and 67% and 56% responded that stress can worsen the condition (p = 0.9999). 50% and 67% correctly responded that exercise may slow the progression of the disease (p = 0.7483), 83% and 89% reported that it does not exclusively affect older individuals (p = 0.9999), 50% and 22% indicated that the sexes are not equally as likely to contract the disease (p = 0.5804) and 83% and 44% concluded that there is a correlation between the disease and depression (p = 0.2867). 33% of both groups had satisfactory knowledge (p = 0.7902), and males boasted an average score of 4.67 while females had a mean score of 4.33 (p = 0.7841) (see Table 3).

DISCUSSION

Only 7% of the surveyed population had a family member affected by the disease. A greater proportion believed they were aware of the disease, and an even greater percentage (53% vs 27%) were actually aware. The results of this survey are in concordance with previous studies (13-17) that young adults are adequately aware.

Table 2. Perceived and actual knowledge

Question Item	n = 15
"I believe I am knowledgeable about Parkinson's disease"	
Agree	4 (27%)
Disagree	5 (33%)
Neutral	6 (40%)
"The cause of Parkinson's disease is unknown"	
True	7 (47%)
False	1 (7%)
Not Sure	7 (47%)
"There is no cure to the disease, only treatments of symptoms"	
True	11 (73%)
False	1 (7%)
Not Sure	3 (20%)
"There is no specific test to diagnose Parkinson's disease"	
True	4 (27%)
False	5 (33%)
Not Sure	6 (40%)
"Stress can worsen the condition"	
True	9 (60%)
False	1 (7%)
Not Sure	5 (33%)
"Exercise may slow the progression of Parkinson's disease"	
True	9 (60%)
False	1 (7%)
Not Sure	5 (33%)
"Parkinson's only affects old people"	
True	0 (0%)
False	13 (87%)
Not Sure	2 (13%)
"Men and women are equally as likely to be affected by Parkinson's"	
True	1 (7%)
False	5 (33%)
Not Sure	9 (60%)
"There is no correlation between Parkinson's and depression"	
True	0 (0%)
False	9 (60%)
Not Sure	6 (40%)
Knowledge Score	
Not Knowledgeable (0-4)	7 (47%)
Satisfactory (5-6)	5 (33%)
Knowledgeable (7-8)	3 (20%)
Mean ± SD	4.47 ± 2.23

Table 3. Perceived and actual knowledge - by subgroups

Question Item	**Under 20 n = 9**	**Over 20 n = 6**	**p-value**
"I believe I am knowledgeable about Parkinson's disease"			0.8127
Agree	3 (33%)	1 (17%)	
Disagree	3 (33%)	2 (33%)	
Neutral	3 (33%)	3 (50%)	
"The cause of Parkinson's disease is unknown"			0.5717
True	4 (44%)	3 (50%)	
False	0 (0%)	1 (17%)	
Not Sure	5 (56%)	2 (33%)	
"There is no cure to the disease, only treatments of symptoms"			0.1181
True	8 (89%)	3 (50%)	
False	1 (11%)	1 (17%)	
Not Sure	0 (0%)	2 (33%)	
"There is no specific test to diagnose Parkinson's disease"			0.9999
True	2 (22%)	2 (33%)	
False	3 (33%)	2 (33%)	
Not Sure	4 (44%)	2 (33%)	
"Stress can worsen the condition"			0.5220
True	6 (67%)	4 (67%)	
False	0 (0%)	1 (17%)	
Not Sure	3 (33%)	1 (17%)	
"Exercise may slow the progression of Parkinson's disease"			0.2335
True	7 (78%)	3 (50%)	
False	1 (11%)	0 (0%)	
Not Sure	1 (11%)	3 (50%)	
"Parkinson's only affects old people"			0.9999
True	0 (0%)	0 (0%)	
False	8 (89%)	5 (83%)	
Not Sure	1 (11%)	1 (17%)	
"Men and women are equally as likely to be affected by Parkinson's"			0.7483
True	1 (11%)	0 (0%)	
False	2 (22%)	3 (50%)	
Not Sure	6 (67%)	3 (50%)	

Table 3. (Continued)

Question Item	**Under 20 n = 9**	**Over 20 n = 6**	**p-value**
"There is no correlation between Parkinson's and depression"			0.1357
True	0 (0%)	0 (0%)	
False	7 (78%)	2 (33%)	
Not Sure	2 (22%)	4 (67%)	
Knowledge Score			
Not Knowledgeable (0-4)	4 (44%)	3 (50%)	0.5385
Satisfactory (5-6)	4 (44%)	1 (17%)	
Knowledgeable (7-8)	1 (11%)	2 (33%)	
Mean ± SD	4.67 ± 1.80	4.17 ± 2.93	0.6869
Question Item	**Males n = 6**	**Females n = 9**	
"I believe I am knowledgeable about Parkinson's disease"			0.9999
Agree	2 (33%)	2 (22%)	
Disagree	2 (33%)	3 (33%)	
Neutral	2 (33%)	4 (44%)	
"The cause of Parkinson's disease is unknown"			0.1678
True	1 (17%)	6 (67%)	
False	1 (17%)	0 (0%)	
Not Sure	4 (67%)	3 (33%)	
"There is no cure to the disease, only treatments of symptoms"			0.7231
True	4 (67%)	7 (78%)	
False	0 (0%)	1 (11%)	
Not Sure	2 (33%)	1 (11%)	
"There is no specific test to diagnose Parkinson's disease"			0.3487
True	3 (50%)	1 (11%)	
False	1 (17%)	4 (44%)	
Not Sure	2 (33%)	4 (44%)	

Question Item	Males n = 6	Females n = 9	
"Stress can worsen the condition"			0.9999
True	4 (67%)	5 (56%)	
False	0 (0%)	1 (11%)	
Not Sure	2 (33%)	3 (33%)	
"Exercise may slow the progression of Parkinson's disease"			0.7483
True	3 (50%)	6 (67%)	
False	1 (17%)	0 (0%)	
Not Sure	2 (33%)	3 (33%)	
"Parkinson's only affects old people"			0.9999
True	0 (0%)	0 (0%)	
False	5 (83%)	8 (89%)	
Not Sure	1 (17%)	1 (11%)	
"Men and women are equally as likely to be affected by Parkinson's"			0.5804
True	0 (0%)	1 (11%)	
False	3 (50%)	2 (22%)	
Not Sure	3 (50%)	6 (67%)	
"There is no correlation between Parkinson's and depression"			0.2867
True	0 (0%)	0 (0%)	
False	5 (83%)	4 (44%)	
Not Sure	1 (17%)	5 (56%)	
Knowledge Score			
Not Knowledgeable (0-4)	2 (33%)	5 (56%)	0.7902
Satisfactory (5-6)	2 (33%)	3 (33%)	
Knowledgeable (7-8)	2 (33%)	1 (11%)	
Mean ± SD	4.67 ± 2.94	4.33 ± 1.80	0.7841

Subgroup analyses showed that neither age nor sex is indicative of knowledge level. However, the sample sizes are noticeably small and the lack of statistical power may explain why no difference was noted. Nevertheless, educational programs should be established to try to increase the awareness of the disease across all subgroups.

This study was not without limitations. The sample size was fairly small, reducing the power of statistical analyses. The survey design also presented the limitation of sampling/response bias.

In conclusion, 53% were knowledgeable about the disease, which is in excess of the 27% who believed they were knowledgeable and also the 7% who had a family member affected by the disease. Educational programs should be setup to increase the awareness of the disease, as there is still room for improvement.

REFERENCES

[1] Parkinson J. An essay on the shaking palsy. London: Whitingham Rowland, 1817.

[2] Polymeropoulos MH, Lavedan C, Leroy E, Ide SE, Dehejia A, Dutra A, et al. Mutation in the α-Synuclein Gene Identified in Families with Parkinson's Disease. Science 1997;276(5321):2045-7.

[3] Global Parkinson's Disease Survey Steering Committee. Factors impacting on quality of life in Parkinson's disease: results from an international survey. Mov Disord 2002;17:60-7.

[4] Chaudhuri KR, Schapira AHV, Martinez-Martin P. The holistic management of Parkinson's using a novel non-motor symptom scale and questionnaire. Adv Clin Neurosci Rehabil 2004;4:20-4.

[5] Aarsland D, Larsen JP, Tandberg E, Laake K. Predictors of nursing home placement in Parkinson's disease: a population-based, prospective study. J Am Geriatr Soc 2000;48:938-42.

[6] Witjas T, Kaphan E, Azulay JP et al. Nonmotor fluctuations in Parkinson's disease: frequent and disabling. Neurology 2002;59:408-13.

[7] Schrag A, Jahanshahi N, Quinn N. What contributes to quality of life in patients with Parkinson's disease? J Neurol Neurosurg Psychiatry 2000;69:308-12.

[8] Findley L, Aujla M, Bain PG et al. Direct economic impact of Parkinson's disease: a research survey in the United Kingdom. Mov Disord 2003;18:1139-45.

[9] Hagell P, Nordling S, Reimer J, Grabowski M, Persson U. Resource use and costs in a Swedish cohort of patients with Parkinson's disease. Mov Disord 2002;17:1213-20.

[10] Pressley JC, Louis ED, Tang MX et al. The impact of comorbid disease and injuries on resource use and expenditures in parkinsonism. Neurology 2003;60:87-93.

[11] Chow R, Borean M, Hollenberg D, Merrick J. How aware/knowledgeable are young adults about Parkinson's disease? J Pain Manage 2019;12(1), in press.

[12] Chow R, Viehweger J, Trasente V, Borean M, Hollenberg D, Lam M, et al. Awareness of Parkinson's disease among young adults in London, Canada. J Pain Manage 2019;12(1), in press.

[13] Ho S, Viehweger J, Trasente V, Ho C, Ng W, Wong M, et al. Awareness of Parkinson's disease among young adults in Toronto, Canada. J Pain Manage 2019;12(1), in press.

[14] Viehweger J, Chow R, Trasente V, Duarte N, Borean M, Hollenberg D, et al. Awareness of Parkinson's disease among young adults in Waterloo, Canada. J Pain Manage 2019;12(1), in press.

[15] Ho S, Viehweger J, Trasente V, Borean M, Hollenberg D, Ferguson T, et al. Awareness of Parkinson's disease among young adults in Halifax, Canada. J Pain Manage 2019;12(1), in press.

[16] Anpalagan T, Chow R, Viehweger J, Trasente V, Borean M, Hollenberg D, et al. Awareness of Parkinson's disease among young adults in Asia. J Pain Manage 2019;12(1), in press.

[17] Viehweger J, Trasente T, Ganguli N, Kang R, Borean M, Hollenberg D, et al. Awareness of Parkinson's disease among young adults in New York State, USA. J Pain Manage 2019;12(1), in press.

[18] Chow R, Borean M, Hollenberg D. Awareness of Parkinson's disease: About the survey instrument. J Pain Manage 2019;12(1), in press.

In: Parkinson's Disease
Editors: Ronald Chow, et al.
ISBN: 978-1-53612-745-4

Chapter 10

AWARENESS OF PARKINSON'S DISEASE AMONG YOUNG ADULTS IN ASIA

Tharani Anpalagan, BMSc(C), Ronald Chow*, BMSc(C), Jaclyn Viehweger, BMSc(C), Victoria Trasente, BA(C), Michael Borean, BMSc(C), Drew Hollenberg, BMSc(C) and Anna Rzepka, BMSc(C)
Infinitas Research Group, London, Ontario, Canada

Numerous studies have been conducted to investigate the awareness of young adults with respect to Parkinson's disease, to determine whether this population is knowledgeable enough to care for affected individuals. These studies all show that young adults are adequately aware, however, there does exist tremendous variation in the awareness level. This variation is noticeable, and seems to be quite significant even among Canadian young adults. It would be interesting to see whether there exists greater variation between Canadian and Asian young adults. The aim of this study was to investigate the awareness level of young adults in Asia.

* Correspondence: Ronald Chow BMSc(C), Infinitas Research Group, London, Ontario, Canada. Email: rchow48@uwo.ca.

A survey was sent out via social media outlets to young adults in Asia (i.e., Taiwan, Singapore). 14 consenting individuals completed the form. 50% are knowledgeable about the disease. When interpreted in light of 21% having a family member affected by the disease and 43% actually believing they are knowledgeable, young adults seem adequately aware of the disease. Nevertheless, education programs should be developed to improve awareness for the entire population, as only a handful (albeit a "satisfactory" amount of people) are knowledgeable. By increasing the knowledge, hopefully this population will be better-equipped to care for affected individuals, as the prevalence of the disease increases.

INTRODUCTION

Numerous studies have been conducted to investigate the awareness of young adults with respect to Parkinson's disease, to determine whether this population is knowledgeable enough to care for affected individuals (1-5). Each study has revealed that young adults are adequately aware about the disease.

The original reported by Chow et al. (2) noted that 54% of young adults in London, Canada, were knowledgeable about the disease. This statistic is lower than the 41% of respondents who believed they were knowledgeable, and 27% who had family members affected by the disease (2).

Ho et al. conducted a study of young adults in Toronto, Canada, and noted that 23% of individuals have a family member afflicted by the disease and also that only 15% believed they were aware of disease. Given the fact that 35% are knowledgeable, the results suggest that they are knowledgeable (3).

A paper about young adults of Waterloo (Canada) by Viehweger et al. (4) concluded that 58% were aware of the disease, 26% believed they were aware of the disease, and 32% had a family member affected by the disease (4). Another study of Halifax (Canada) young adults noted that 40% were knowledgeable, while only 27% believed they were knowledgeable and 7% had family members affected by the disease (5).

These studies all show that young adults are adequately aware, however, there does exist tremendous variation in the awareness level. This variation is noticeable, and seems to be quite significant even among Canadian young adults. It would be interesting to see whether there exists greater variation between Canadian and Asian young adults. The aim of this study was to investigate the awareness level of young adults in Asia.

STUDY

A survey was sent out via social media outlets to young adults in Asia (i.e., Taiwan, Singapore). The survey was voluntary. The consent form on the first page acknowledged that there are no benefits/costs to participants, and required participants to consent to the study. The second page collected demographic information and the third page was used to determine the actual and perceived awareness of Parkinson's disease (6).

Descriptive statistics were used to disclose participant demographics, and the number of correct/incorrect answers. Fisher exact tests were used to determine whether there was a difference in categorical questions between age groups (under and over 20 years old), gender groups (males and females), familial ties (affected and not affected by Parkinson's disease) and the frequency of visiting their family members (less than and over 10 visits a year). ANOVA procedures compared the average number of correct answers between the subgroups. All analyses were conducted using the Statistical Analysis Software (SAS Version 9.4 for Windows) (6).

FINDINGS

14 consenting individuals completed the form. 5 (36%) were over 22 years old, and the remaining 9 were split evenly between the age cohorts of under 18 years old (21%), 18-19 years old (21%), and 20-22 years old (21%). 5 (36%) declared that they are males, 7 were females (50%) and the remaining (14%) did not identify. The majority of young adults (79%) do not have a family member affected by the disease; of the 21% affected, 33% visited less than 3 times a year and 67% visited more than 20 times a year (see Table 1).

Table 1. Demographics

Demographic	**n = 14**
Age Group	
Under 18 years old	3 (21%)
18-19 years old	3 (21%)
20-22 years old	3 (21%)
Over 22 years old	5 (36%)
Sex	
Male	5 (36%)
Female	7 (50%)
Prefer not to say	2 (14%)
Family member affected by Parkinson's disease	
Yes	3 (21%)
No	11 (79%)
Number of visits to Parkinson's family member a year (n=3)	
Less than 3	1 (33%)
3-10	0 (0%)
10-20	0 (0%)
20+	2 (67%)

Table 2. Perceived and actual knowledge

Question Item	n = 14
"I believe I am knowledgeable about Parkinson's disease"	
Agree	6 (43%)
Disagree	3 (21%)
Neutral	5 (36%)
"The cause of Parkinson's disease is unknown"	
True	7 (50%)
False	1 (7%)
Not Sure	6 (43%)
"There is no cure to the disease, only treatments of symptoms"	
True	10 (71%)
False	0 (0%)
Not Sure	4 (29%)
"There is no specific test to diagnose Parkinson's disease"	
True	3 (21%)
False	3 (21%)
Not Sure	8 (57%)
"Stress can worsen the condition"	
True	9 (64%)
False	0 (0%)
Not Sure	5 (36%)
"Exercise may slow the progression of Parkinson's disease"	
True	10 (71%)
False	0 (0%)
Not Sure	4 (29%)
"Parkinson's only affects old people"	
True	1 (7%)
False	10 (71%)
Not Sure	3 (21%)
"Men and women are equally as likely to be affected by Parkinson's"	
True	5 (36%)
False	3 (21%)
Not Sure	6 (43%)

Table 2. (Continued)

Question Item	**n = 14**
"There is no correlation between Parkinson's and depression"	
True	2 (14%)
False	4 (29%)
Not Sure	8 (57%)
Knowledge Score	
Not Knowledgeable (0-4)	7 (50%)
Satisfactory (5-6)	4 (29%)
Knowledgeable (7-8)	3 (21%)
Mean ± SD	4.00 ± 2.45

43% of young adults believed they were knowledgeable about the disease. 50% correctly noted that Parkinson's disease has an unknown cause, 71% noted that there is no cure to the disease, and 21% answered that there is no diagnostic test. 64% concluded that stress can worsen the condition, 71% indicated that exercise may slow the progression, 71% reported that it does not exclusively affect older individuals, 21% correctly informed that it does not have an equally likelihood of affecting men and women, and 29% concluded that there is a correlation between Parkinson's and depression. Overall, 21% were knowledgeable and 29% had satisfactory knowledge; the average score was 4.00 out of 8 (see Table 2).

Subgroup analysis by age revealed that there exists no difference in perceived or actual awareness between the two groups. 50% and 38% of the younger and older cohorts, respectively, believed they were knowledgeable about the disease (p=0.5005). 50% of both remarked that the cause is unknown (p=0.9999), 67% and 75% noted that there is no cure to the disease (p=0.9999), 17% and 25% indicated that there does not exist a diagnostic test, 67% and 63% reported that stress can worsen the condition (p=0.9999), 67% and 75% reported that exercise may slow the progression of the disease (p=0.9999), 67% and 75%

correctly identified that it does not only affect old people (p=0.7483), 17% and 25% noted that men and women are not equally as likely to be affected (p=0.9999), and 50% and 17% noted that there is a correlation between the disease and depression. 50% of both groups were deemed not knowledgeable based on the overall score (p=0.9999), and both groups averaged scores of 4.00 out of 8 (p=0.9999) (see Table 3).

Table 3. Perceived and actual knowledge - by subgroups

Question Item	Under 20 n = 6	Over 20 n = 8	p-value
"I believe I am knowledgeable about Parkinson's disease"			0.5005
Agree	3 (50%)	3 (38%)	
Disagree	2 (33%)	1 (13%)	
Neutral	1 (17%)	4 (50%)	
"The cause of Parkinson's disease is unknown"			0.9999
True	3 (50%)	4 (50%)	
False	0 (0%)	1 (13%)	
Not Sure	3 (50%)	3 (38%)	
"There is no cure to the disease, only treatments of symptoms"			0.9999
True	4 (67%)	6 (75%)	
False	0 (0%)	0 (0%)	
Not Sure	2 (33%)	2 (25%)	
"There is no specific test to diagnose Parkinson's disease"			0.7902
True	1 (17%)	2 (25%)	
False	2 (33%)	1 (13%)	
Not Sure	3 (50%)	5 (63%)	
"Stress can worsen the condition"			0.9999
True	4 (67%)	5 (63%)	
False	0 (0%)	0 (0%)	
Not Sure	2 (33%)	3 (38%)	

Table 3. (Continued)

Question Item	Under 20 n = 6	Over 20 n = 8	p-value
"Exercise may slow the progression of Parkinson's disease"			0.9999
True	4 (67%)	6 (75%)	
False	0 (0%)	0 (0%)	
Not Sure	2 (33%)	2 (25%)	
"Parkinson's only affects old people"			0.7483
True	1 (17%)	0 (0%)	
False	4 (67%)	6 (75%)	
Not Sure	1 (17%)	2 (25%)	
"Men and women are equally as likely to be affected by Parkinson's"			0.9999
True	2 (33%)	3 (38%)	
False	1 (17%)	2 (25%)	
Not Sure	3 (50%)	3 (38%)	
"There is no correlation between Parkinson's and depression"			0.4499
True	1 (17%)	1 (17%)	
False	3 (50%)	1 (17%)	
Not Sure	2 (33%)	6 (75%)	
Knowledge Score			
Not Knowledgeable (0-4)	3 (50%)	4 (50%)	0.9999
Satisfactory (5-6)	2 (33%)	2 (25%)	
Knowledgeable (7-8)	1 (17%)	2 (25%)	
Mean ± SD	4.00 ± 2.60	4.00 ± 2.51	0.9999
Question Item	**Males n = 5**	**Females n = 7**	
"I believe I am knowledgeable about Parkinson's disease"			0.7727
Agree	1 (20%)	3 (43%)	
Disagree	2 (40%)	1 (14%)	
Neutral	2 (40%)	3 (43%)	

Question Item	Males n = 5	Females n = 7	
"The cause of Parkinson's disease is unknown"			0.1477
True	1 (20%)	5 (71%)	
False	1 (20%)	0 (0%)	
Not Sure	3 (60%)	2 (29%)	
"There is no cure to the disease, only treatments of symptoms"			0.5227
True	3 (60%)	6 (86%)	
False	0 (0%)	0 (0%)	
Not Sure	2 (40%)	1 (14%)	
"There is no specific test to diagnose Parkinson's disease"			0.9999
True	1 (20%)	1 (14%)	
False	1 (20%)	2 (29%)	
Not Sure	3 (60%)	4 (57%)	
"Stress can worsen the condition"			0.0101
True	1 (20%)	7 (100%)	
False	0 (0%)	0 (0%)	
Not Sure	4 (80%)	0 (0%)	
"Exercise may slow the progression of Parkinson's disease"			0.5227
True	3 (60%)	6 (86%)	
False	0 (0%)	0 (0%)	
Not Sure	2 (40%)	1 (14%)	
"Parkinson's only affects old people"			0.1515
True	0 (0%)	0 (0%)	
False	3 (60%)	7 (100%)	
Not Sure	2 (40%)	0 (0%)	
"Men and women are equally as likely to be affected by Parkinson's"			0.7727
True	1 (20%)	3 (43%)	
False	1 (20%)	2 (29%)	
Not Sure	3 (60%)	2 (29%)	

Table 3. (Continued)

Question Item	**Males** **n = 5**	**Females** **n = 7**	
"There is no correlation between Parkinson's and depression"			0.9999
True	0 (0%)	1 (14%)	
False	2 (40%)	2 (29%)	
Not Sure	3 (60%)	4 (57%)	
Knowledge Score			
Not Knowledgeable (0-4)	4 (80%)	2 (29%)	0.2121
Satisfactory (5-6)	0 (0%)	3 (43%)	
Knowledgeable (7-8)	1 (20%)	2 (29%)	
Mean ± SD	3.00 ± 2.65	5.14 ± 1.77	0.1223
Question Item	**Affected** **n = 3**	**Unaffected** **n = 11**	
"I believe I am knowledgeable about Parkinson's disease"			0.3819
Agree	2 (67%)	4 (36%)	
Disagree	1 (33%)	2 (18%)	
Neutral	0 (0%)	5 (45%)	
"The cause of Parkinson's disease is unknown"			0.6538
True	1 (33%)	6 (55%)	
False	0 (0%)	1 (9%)	
Not Sure	2 (67%)	4 (36%)	
"There is no cure to the disease, only treatments of symptoms"			0.5055
True	1 (33%)	8 (73%)	
False	0 (0%)	0 (0%)	
Not Sure	2 (67%)	3 (27%)	
"There is no specific test to diagnose Parkinson's disease"			0.9999
True	1 (33%)	2 (18%)	
False	0 (0%)	3 (27%)	
Not Sure	2 (67%)	6 (55%)	

Question Item	**Affected** **n = 3**	**Unaffected** **n = 11**	
"Stress can worsen the condition"			0.5055
True	1 (33%)	8 (73%)	
False	0 (0%)	0 (0%)	
Not Sure	2 (67%)	3 (27%)	
"Exercise may slow the progression of Parkinson's disease"			0.1758
True	1 (33%)	9 (82%)	
False	0 (0%)	0 (0%)	
Not Sure	2 (67%)	2 (18%)	
"Parkinson's only affects old people"			0.0934
True	1 (33%)	0 (0%)	
False	1 (33%)	9 (82%)	
Not Sure	1 (33%)	2 (18%)	
"Men and women are equally as likely to be affected by Parkinson's"			0.7527
True	1 (33%)	4 (36%)	
False	0 (0%)	3 (27%)	
Not Sure	2 (67%)	4 (36%)	
"There is no correlation between Parkinson's and depression"			0.6923
True	1 (33%)	1 (9%)	
False	1 (33%)	3 (27%)	
Not Sure	1 (33%)	7 (64%)	
Knowledge Score			
Not Knowledgeable (0-4)	2 (67%)	5 (45%)	0.9999
Satisfactory (5-6)	1 (33%)	3 (27%)	
Knowledgeable (7-8)	0 (0%)	3 (27%)	
Mean ± SD	2.33 ± 2.52	4.45 ± 2.34	0.1949

There was also no difference in overall responses between males and females. Females more often correctly answered that stress can worsen the condition (100%) compared to males (20%) (p=0.0101). 20% and 43% of males and females, respectively, believed they were knowledgeable (p=0.7727). 20% and 71% noted that there is no cure (p=0.1477), 60% and 86% noted that there is no cure (p=0.5227), and 20% and 14% responded that there is no diagnostic test (p=0.9999). 60% and 86% noted that exercise may slow the progression of the disease (p=0.5227), 60% and 100% answered that it does not only affect old people (p=0.1515), 20% and 43% incorrectly answered that men and women share similar likelihoods of contracting the disease (p=0.7727), and 40% and 29% noted that there is a correlation between the disease and depression (p=0.9999). Overall, 20% and 29% were knowledgeable (p=0.2121), with average scores for the two groups being 3.00 and 5.14 (p=0.1223) (see Table 3).

Responses were similar for those with a family affected and those without a family member affected by the disease. 67% and 36% of those affected and unaffected, respectively, believed they were knowledgeable (p=0.3819). 33% and 55% of the same groups indicated that the cause is unknown (p=0.6538), 33% and 73% noted that there is no cure to the disease (p=0.5055), 33% and 18% answered that there is no specific diagnostic test (p=0.9999), 33% and 73% concluded that stress can worsen the condition (p=0.5055), 33% and 82% identified that exercise may slow the progression (p=0.1758) and 33% and 82% answered that it does not only affect old people (p=0.0934). 33% and 36% incorrectly answered that men and women are equally as likely to be affected by the disease (p=0.7527), and 33% and 9% incorrectly noted that there is no correlation between Parkinson's and depression (p=0.6923). 67% and 45% were deemed not knowledgeable (p=0.9999), and the average scores were 2.33 and 43.45, respectively (p=0.1949) (see Table 3).

DISCUSSION

The results herein reveal that 50% are knowledgeable about the disease, and only 21% and 43% have a family member affected and believed they were knowledgeable, respectively. These statistics indicate that young adults in Asia seem to be adequately aware of the disease, which is in line with other studies (2-5).

Our study also shows that there is no difference in responses between cohorts. It is important to note that our study did not a small sample size and hence cohort analyses had extremely limited statistical power - future studies should re-examine the responses with greater statistical power. Nevertheless, education programs should be developed to improve awareness for the entire population, as only a handful (albeit a "satisfactory" amount of people) are knowledgeable. By increasing the knowledge, hopefully this population will be better-equipped to care for affected individuals, as the prevalence of the disease increases (1).

This study was not without limitations. Due to the nature of the study design, there exists the possibility of a response and sampling bias. Additionally, the sample size restricted the power of subgroup analyses.

In conclusion, 50% are knowledgeable about the disease. When interpreted in light of 21% having a family member affected by the disease and 43% actually believing they are knowledgeable, young adults seem adequately aware of the disease. Nevertheless, education programs should be developed to improve awareness for the entire population, as only a handful (albeit a "satisfactory" amount of people) are knowledgeable. By increasing the knowledge, hopefully this population will be better-equipped to care for affected individuals, as the prevalence of the disease increases.

References

[1] Chow R, Borean M, Hollenberg D, Merrick J. How aware/knowledgeable are young adults about Parkinson's disease? J Pain Manage 2019;12(1), in press.

[2] Chow R, Viehweger J, Trasente V, Borean M, Hollenberg D, Lam M, et al. Awareness of Parkinson's disease among young adults in London, Canada. J Pain Manage 2019;12(1), in press.

[3] Ho S, Viehweger J, Trasente V, Ho C, Ng W, Wong M et al. Awareness of Parkinson's disease among young adults in Toronto, Canada. J Pain Manage 2019;12(1), in press.

[4] Viehweger J, Chow R, Trasente V, Duarte N, Borean M, Hollenberg D et al. Awareness of Parkinson's disease among young adults in Waterloo, Canada. J Pain Manage 2019;12(1), in press.

[5] Ho S, Viehweger J, Trasente V, Borean M, Hollenberg D, Ferguson T et al. Awareness of Parkinson's disease among young adults in Halifax, Canada. J Pain Manage 2019;12(1), in press.

[6] Chow R, Borean M, Hollenberg D. Awareness of Parkinson's disease: About the survey instrument. J Pain Manage 2019;12(1), in press.

SECTION THREE: OVERALL AWARENESS

In: Parkinson's Disease
Editors: Ronald Chow, et al.
ISBN: 978-1-53612-745-4

Chapter 11

AWARENESS OF PARKINSON'S DISEASE AMONG YOUNG ADULTS: A META-ANALYSIS

Ronald Chow**, BMSc(C)
and Jaclyn Viehweger, BMSc(C)
Infinitas Research Group, London, Ontario, Canada

Many studies have been conducted among young adults across the world, using a survey, to assess the knowledge of this cohort. The aim of this chapter is to summarize the studies documenting the awareness of Parkinson's disease. For each endpoint, the values for the respective endpoints from prior studies were summed. Descriptive statistics were used to portray the summed demographics of respondents, and Fisher-exact tests were carried out to statistically test whether there was a difference in subgroups with respect to categorical questions. 50% were knowledgeable about the disease. This statistic is in excess of the 21% who had family members with the disease and the 30% who believed they were knowledgeable. The results indicate that young adults are adequately aware of the disease, and also that there is plenty of room to increase the awareness among the young adult population through educational programs.

---

* Correspondence: Ronald Chow BMSc(C), Infinitas Research Group, London, Ontario, Canada. Email: rchow48@uwo.ca.

Introduction

The disease that James Parkinson described originally in 1817, Parkinson's disease, is a neurodegenerative disease with debilitating symptoms (1-2). The disabling symptoms can be broadly classified into two categories - motor (resting tremor, muscular rigidity, bradykinesia) and nonmotor (quality of life, depression, sleep disturbances) symptoms (3-12).

There is no cure for the disease, and only treatments for symptoms (13). Hence, to improve standard of care for affected patients, it has been proposed that increased knowledge and awareness by caregivers could provide more holistic and individualized care (13). Many studies have been conducted among young adults across the world, using a survey (14), to assess the knowledge of this cohort (15-22). The aim of this review is to summarize the studies documenting the awareness.

Our study

For each endpoint, the values for the respective endpoints from prior studies were summed. Descriptive statistics were used to portray the summed demographics of respondents, and Fisher-exact tests were carried out to statistically test whether there was a difference in subgroups with respect to categorical questions.

Findings

Across the eight studies included in this meta-analysis, the total sample size was 167 participants (see Table 1). Individual study sample sizes ranged from 13 by Viehweger et al. about young adults in New York State (20) to 41 by Chow et al. about young adults in London (15). One study was conducted in Ireland (21), another in United States of America (20), a third in Asia (19) and the remaining in Canada (15-18,22) (see Table 1).

The majority of participants (59%) were between 18 and 19 years old, while 23% were between 20 and 22 years old, 12% over 22 years old, and 7% under 18 years old. Three-quarters were female, while 23% were male and 2% did not remark which sex they were. 21% of the population had a family member affected by the disease, to their knowledge. Of the 21%, 40% visited their family member more than 20 times a year, 20% between 10-20 times a year, 14% between 3 and 10, and 26% less than 3 a year (see Table 2).

30% believed they were knowledgeable about the disease. 38% remarked that the cause of the disease is unknown, 83% noted that there is no cure to the disease, 23% concluded that there is no diagnostic test, 69% answered that stress can worsen the condition, and 56% indicated that exercise may slow the progression of the disease. 90% noted that Parkinson's does not solely affect old people, 33% remarked that the two sexes are not equally as likely to be affected, and 50% responded that there is a correlation between the disease and depression. 50% were deemed not knowledgeable, 34% had satisfactory knowledge, and 16% were knowledgeable (see Table 3).

Table 1. Included Studies

Study	Region	Sample Size
Chow et al. (15)	London, Canada	41
Ho et al. (16)	Toronto, Canada	26
Viehweger et al. (17)	Waterloo, Canada	19
Ho et al. (18)	Halifax, Canada	15
Anpalagan et al. (19)	Asia	14
Viehweger et al. (20)	New York State, United States of America	13
Hollenberg et al. (21)	Dublin, Ireland	15
Borean et al. (22)	Kingston, Canada	24

Table 2. Demographics

Demographic	n = 167
Age Group	
Under 18 years old	11 (7%)
18-19 years old	98 (59%)
20-22 years old	38 (23%)
Over 22 years old	20 (12%)
Sex	
Male	39 (23%)
Female	125 (75%)
Prefer not to say	3 (2%)
Family member affected by Parkinson's disease	
Yes	35 (21%)
No	132 (79%)
Number of visits to Parkinson's family member a year (n = 35)	
Less than 3	9 (26%)
3-10	5 (14%)
10-20	7 (20%)
20+	14 (40%)

Table 3. Perceived and actual knowledge

Question Item	n = 167
"I believe I am knowledgeable about Parkinson's disease"	
Agree	50 (30%)
Disagree	49 (29%)
Neutral	68 (41%)
"The cause of Parkinson's disease is unknown"	
True	63 (38%)
False	31 (19%)
Not Sure	73 (44%)
"There is no cure to the disease, only treatments of symptoms"	
True	138 (83%)
False	5 (3%)
Not Sure	24 (15%)
"There is no specific test to diagnose Parkinson's disease"	
True	39 (23%)
False	64 (38%)
Not Sure	64 (38%)

Question Item	n = 167
"Stress can worsen the condition"	
True	116 (69%)
False	6 (4%)
Not Sure	45 (27%)
"Exercise may slow the progression of Parkinson's disease"	
True	94 (56%)
False	14 (8%)
Not Sure	59 (35%)
"Parkinson's only affects old people"	
True	4 (2%)
False	150 (90%)
Not Sure	13 (8%)
"Men and women are equally as likely to be affected by	
Parkinson's"	36 (22%)
True	55 (33%)
False	76 (46%)
Not Sure	
"There is no correlation between Parkinson's and depression"	
Truc	11 (7%)
False	84 (50%)
Not Sure	72 (43%)
Knowledge Score	
Not Knowledgeable (0-4)	84 (50%)
Satisfactory (5-6)	57 (34%)
Knowledgeable (7-8)	26 (16%)

A total of 109 participants were under 20 years old, and 58 were over 20 years old. There was no difference in perceived awareness and overall awareness. 29% and 31% of the two groups, respectively, believed they were knowledgeable about the disease ($p = 0.4983$). 35% and 33% had satisfactory knowledge ($p = 0.6848$). Those under 20 years old were more likely to respond correctly that stress can worsen the condition (72% vs 66%; $p = 0.0197$). There were no difference in other questions: cause of disease ($p - 0.1425$), treatment of symptoms ($p = 0.2988$), diagnostic test ($p = 0.8369$), exercise and the disease ($p = 0.6187$), the affected population ($p = 0.4149$), the chances of males/females contracting the disease (p = 0.8133) and the correlation between Parkinson's and depression (p = 0.3921) (see Table 4).

Table 4. Perceived and actual knowledge - by subgroups

Question Item	**Under 20** **n = 109**	**Over 20** **n = 58**	**p-value**
"I believe I am knowledgeable about Parkinson's disease"			0.4983
Agree	32 (29%)	18 (31%)	
Disagree	38 (35%)	15 (26%)	
Neutral	39 (36%)	25 (43%)	
"The cause of Parkinson's disease is unknown"			0.1425
True	36 (33%)	27 (47%)	
False	21 (19%)	12 (21%)	
Not Sure	52 (48%)	19 (33%)	
"There is no cure to the disease, only treatments of symptoms"			0.2988
True	91 (83%)	46 (79%)	
False	2 (2%)	4 (7%)	
Not Sure	16 (15%)	8 (14%)	
"There is no specific test to diagnose Parkinson's disease"			0.8369
True	24 (22%)	15 (26%)	
False	43 (39%)	21 (36%)	
Not Sure	42 (39%)	22 (38%)	
"Stress can worsen the condition"			0.0197
True	78 (72%)	38 (66%)	
False	1 (1%)	6 (10%)	
Not Sure	30 (28%)	14 (24%)	
"Exercise may slow the progression of Parkinson's disease"			0.6187
True	61 (56%)	34 (59%)	
False	11 (11%)	3 (5%)	
Not Sure	37 (34%)	21 (36%)	
"Parkinson's only affects old people"			0.4149
True	4 (4%)	0 (0%)	
False	96 (88%)	54 (93%)	
Not Sure	9 (8%)	4 (7%)	

Question Item	Under 20 n = 109	Over 20 n = 58	p-value
"Men and women are equally as likely to be affected by Parkinson's"			0.8133
True	22 (20%)	14 (24%)	
False	36 (33%)	19 (33%)	
Not Sure	51 (47%)	25 (43%)	
"There is no correlation between Parkinson's and depression"			0.3921
True	6 (6%)	5 (9%)	
False	60 (55%)	26 (45%)	
Not Sure	43 (39%)	27 (47%)	
Knowledge Score			0.6848
Not Knowledgeable (0-4)	56 (51%)	28 (48%)	
Satisfactory (5-6)	38 (35%)	19 (33%)	
Knowledgeable (7-8)	15 (14%)	11 (19%)	
Question Item	**Males n = 36**	**Females n = 128**	
"I believe I am knowledgeable about Parkinson's disease"			0.5232
Agree	11 (31%)	36 (28%)	
Disagree	8 (22%)	41 (32%)	
Neutral	17 (47%)	51 (40%)	
"The cause of Parkinson's disease is unknown"			0.2358
True	10 (28%)	51 (40%)	
False	10 (28%)	21 (16%)	
Not Sure	16 (44%)	56 (44%)	
"There is no cure to the disease, only treatments of symptoms"			0.6974
True	30 (83%)	106 (83%)	
False	0 (0%)	5 (4%)	
Not Sure	6 (17%)	17 (13%)	
"There is no specific test to diagnose Parkinson's disease"			0.6354
True	10 (28%)	27 (21%)	
False	14 (39%)	50 (39%)	
Not Sure	12 (33%)	51 (40%)	

Table 4. (Continued)

Question Item	Males n = 36	Females n = 128	
"Stress can worsen the condition"			0.1222
True	22 (61%)	92 (72%)	
False	0 (0%)	6 (5%)	
Not Sure	14 (39%)	30 (23%)	
"Exercise may slow the progression of Parkinson's disease"			0.3622
True	24 (67%)	68 (53%)	
False	2 (6%)	11 (9%)	
Not Sure	10 (28%)	49 (38%)	
"Parkinson's only affects old people"			0.1100
True	1 (3%)	1 (1%)	
False	30 (83%)	120 (94%)	
Not Sure	5 (14%)	7 (5%)	
"Men and women are equally as likely to be affected by Parkinson's"			0.4732
True	8 (22%)	26 (20%)	
False	9 (25%)	46 (36%)	
Not Sure	19 (53%)	56 (44%)	
"There is no correlation between Parkinson's and depression"			0.9517
True	2 (6%)	7 (5%)	
False	19 (53%)	64 (50%)	
Not Sure	15 (42%)	57 (45%)	
Knowledge Score			0.0961
Not Knowledgeable (0-4)	21 (58%)	62 (48%)	
Satisfactory (5-6)	7 (19%)	48 (38%)	
Knowledgeable (7-8)	8 (22%)	18 (14%)	
Question Item	**Affected n = 32**	**Unaffected n = 92**	
"I believe I am knowledgeable about Parkinson's disease"			0.5041
Agree	13 (41%)	27 (29%)	
Disagree	9 (28%)	30 (33%)	
Neutral	10 (31%)	35 (38%)	

Question Item	Affected n = 32	Unaffected n = 92	
"The cause of Parkinson's disease is unknown"			0.6983
True	11 (34%)	34 (37%)	
False	9 (28%)	19 (21%)	
Not Sure	12 (38%)	39 (42%)	
"There is no cure to the disease, only treatments of symptoms"			0.3300
True	30 (94%)	76 (83%)	
False	0 (0%)	2 (2%)	
Not Sure	2 (6%)	14 (15%)	
"There is no specific test to diagnose Parkinson's disease"			0.0564
True	10 (31%)	20 (22%)	
False	7 (22%)	42 (46%)	
Not Sure	15 (47%)	30 (33%)	
"Stress can worsen the condition"			0.9999
True	24 (75%)	69 (75%)	
False	1 (3%)	2 (2%)	
Not Sure	7 (22%)	21 (23%)	
"Exercise may slow the progression of Parkinson's disease"			0.7509
True	17 (53%)	55 (60%)	
False	3 (9%)	9 (10%)	
Not Sure	12 (38%)	28 (30%)	
"Parkinson's only affects old people"			0.1740
True	2 (6%)	1 (1%)	
False	29 (91%)	83 (90%)	
Not Sure	1 (3%)	8 (9%)	
"Men and women are equally as likely to be affected by Parkinson's"			0.6787
True	8 (25%)	22 (24%)	
False	9 (28%)	34 (37%)	
Not Sure	15 (47%)	36 (39%)	
"There is no correlation between Parkinson's and depression"			0.1688
True	2 (6%)	6 (7%)	
False	20 (63%)	40 (43%)	
Not Sure	10 (31%)	46 (50%)	

Table 4. (Continued)

Question Item	Affected n = 32	Unaffected n = 92	
Knowledge Score			0.9607
Not Knowledgeable (0-4)	15 (47%)	46 (50%)	
Satisfactory (5-6)	12 (38%)	31 (34%)	
Knowledgeable (7-8)	5 (16%)	15 (16%)	
Question Item	**Less than 10 visits n = 12**	**More than 10 visits n = 17**	
"I believe I am knowledgeable about Parkinson's disease"			0.8545
Agree	5 (42%)	6 (35%)	
Disagree	1 (8%)	1 (6%)	
Neutral	6 (50%)	10 (59%)	
"The cause of Parkinson's disease is unknown"			0.5748
True	3 (25%)	7 (41%)	
False	5 (42%)	4 (24%)	
Not Sure	4 (33%)	6 (35%)	
"There is no cure to the disease, only treatments of symptoms"			0.9999
True	12 (100%)	17 (100%)	
False	0 (0%)	0 (0%)	
Not Sure	0 (0%)	0 (0%)	
"There is no specific test to diagnose Parkinson's disease"			0.1355
True	6 (50%)	3 (18%)	
False	3 (25%)	4 (24%)	
Not Sure	3 (25%)	10 (59%)	
"Stress can worsen the condition"			0.3544
True	11 (92%)	12 (71%)	
False	0 (0%)	0 (0%)	
Not Sure	1 (8%)	5 (29%)	
"Exercise may slow the progression of Parkinson's disease"			0.5580
True	7 (58%)	9 (53%)	
False	2 (17%)	1 (6%)	
Not Sure	3 (25%)	7 (41%)	

Question Item	**Less than 10 visits n = 12**	**More than 10 visits n = 17**	
"Parkinson's only affects old people"			0.3138
True	1 (8%)	0 (0%)	
False	11 (92%)	17 (100%)	
Not Sure	0 (0%)	0 (0%)	
"Men and women are equally as likely to be affected by Parkinson's"			0.5674
True	4 (33%)	3 (18%)	
False	4 (33%)	5 (29%)	
Not Sure	4 (3%)	9 (53%)	
"There is no correlation between Parkinson's and depression"			0.2341
True	1 (8%)	0 (0%)	
False	9 (75%)	10 (59%)	
Not Sure	2 (17%)	7 (41%)	
Knowledge Score			0.6181
Not Knowledgeable (0-4)	4 (33%)	9 (53%)	
Satisfactory (5-6)	6 (50%)	5 (29%)	
Knowledgeable (7-8)	2 (17%)	3 (18%)	

There was also no difference in perceived and overall awareness between males (n = 36) and females (n = 128). 31% and 28% of the two sexes, respectively, believed they were knowledgeable about the disease (p = 0.5232). 28% and 40% noted that there is no known cause, 83% of both groups indicated that there is no cure, and 28% and 21% answered that there is no diagnostic test (p = 0.6354). The fact that stress can worsen the condition was acknowledged by 61% and 72% (p = 0.1222), that exercise may slow the progression by 67% and 53% (p = 0.3622), that it does not only affect people by 83% and 94% (p = 0.1100), that males and females are not equally likely to be affected by the disease by 25% and 36% (p = 0.4732), and that there is a correlation between the disease and depression by 53% and 50% (p – 0.9517). 22% of males were knowledgeable and 14% of females were considered knowledgeable (p = 0.0961) (see Table 4).

Between the 32 individuals with family members affected by the disease and 92 without affected family members, there was no difference in knowledge between the two cohorts. 41% and 29% of those affected and unaffected, respectively, noted that they were knowledgeable about the disease ($p = 0.5041$). 34% and 37% answered that the cause is unknown ($p = 0.6983$), 94% and 83% indicated that there is no cure to the disease ($p = 0.3300$), 31% and 21% noted that there is no diagnostic test ($p = 0.0564$), and 75% of both groups concluded that stress can worsen the condition ($p = 0.9999$). 53% and 60% answered that exercise may slow the progression of the disease ($p = 0.7509$), 91% and 90% noted that it affects individuals other than elderlies ($p = 0.1740$), 28% and 37% concluded that it does not have an equal likelihood of affecting males and females ($p = 0.6787$), and 63% and 43% indicated that there is a correlation between the disease and depression ($p = 0.1688$). 47% and 50% were not knowledgeable, overall ($p = 0.9607$) (see table 4).

The fourth subgroup analysis between those who visit their family members more than and less than 10 times a year also found no statistical difference in awareness. 42% and 35% believed they were knowledgeable about the disease ($p = 0.8545$). 25% and 41% answered that there is no known cause ($p = 0.5748$), 100% of both noted that there is no cure ($p = 0.9999$), 50% and 18% concluded that there is no diagnostic test ($p = 0.1355$), 92% and 71% indicated that stress can worsen the condition ($p = 0.3544$), 58% and 53% responded that exercise may slow the progression ($p = 0.5580$), 92% and 100% answered that it does not only affect elderlies ($p = 0.3138$), 33% and 29% noted that men and women are not equally as likely to be affected by the disease ($p = 0.5674$) and 75% and 59% noted that there is a correlation between the disease and depression ($p = 0.2341$). 17% and 18% of the two groups were knowledgeable ($p = 0.6181$) (see Table 4).

DISCUSSION

Half of the respondents had either satisfactory knowledge or were knowledgeable about the disease. When interpreted in light of the fact that 21% had a family member affected by the disease and that 30% believed they were aware of the disease, it seems that young adults are adequately aware of the disease. Nevertheless, 1 in 2 young adults still are not knowledgeable about the disease - education programs should be established to increase the awareness of the disease.

Subgroup analyses showed that no specific demographic group was more knowledgeable or perceived themselves to be more knowledgeable, when compared to the other group. All subgroups were also more aware than they perceived themselves to be. Such information is comforting, in the sense that those who have little exposure to the disease also have the same knowledge level as those with immense exposure to the disease through a related family member. However, it may also be discouraging to see that those who regularly visit their family members are not more knowledgeable about the disease than those who rarely visit a family member. Such a finding seems to support the need for educational programs to increase the awareness of the disease, as mere exposure does not seem to increase the knowledge of young adults.

In conclusion, 50% of participants were knowledgeable about the disease. This statistic is in excess of the 21% who had family members with the disease and the 30% who believed they were knowledgeable. The results indicate that young adults are adequately aware of the disease, and also that there is plenty of room to increase the awareness among the young adult population through educational programs.

ACKNOWLEDGMENTS

We would like to thank Michael Borean, Drew Hollenberg, Tharani Anpalagan, Anna Rzepka and Victoria Trasente in their support of this meta-analysis.

REFERENCES

[1] Parkinson J. An essay on the shaking palsy. London: Whitingham Rowland, 1817.

[2] Polymeropoulos MH, Lavedan C, Leroy E, Ide SE, Dehejia A, Dutra A, et al. Mutation in the α-synuclein gene identified in families with Parkinson's disease. Science 1997;276(5321):2045-7.

[3] Hughes AJ, Daniel SE, Kilford L, Lees AJ. Accuracy of clinical diagnosis of idiopathic Parkinson's disease: a clinico-pathological study of 100 cases. J Neurol Neurosurg Psychiatry 1992;55:181-4.

[4] Fahn S, Elton RL, UPDRS Development Committee. Unified Parkinson's disease rating scale. In: Fahn S, Marsden CD, Calne D, Goldstein M, eds. Recent developments in Parkinson's disease. Florham Park, NJ: MacMillan Healthcare Information, 1987:153-63.

[5] Global Parkinson's Disease Survey Steering Committee. Factors impacting on quality of life in Parkinson's disease: results from an international survey. Mov Disord 2002;17:60-7.

[6] Chaudhuri KR, Schapira AHV, Martinez-Martin P. The holistic management of Parkinson's using a novel non-motor symptom scale and questionnaire. Adv Clin Neurosci Rehabil 2004;4:20-4.

[7] Aarsland D, Larsen JP, Tandberg E, Laake K. Predictors of nursing home placement in Parkinson's disease: a population-based, prospective study. J Am Geriatr Soc 2000;48:938-42.

[8] Witjas T, Kaphan E, Azulay JP, Blin O, Ceccaldi M, Pouget J, et al. Nonmotor fluctuations in Parkinson's disease: frequent and disabling. Neurology 2002;59:408-13.

[9] Schrag A, Jahanshahi N, Quinn N. What contributes to quality of life in patients with Parkinson's disease? J Neurol Neurosurg Psychiatry 2000;69:308-12.

[10] Findley L, Aujla M, Bain PG, Baker M, Beech C, Bowman C, et al. Direct economic impact of Parkinson's disease: a research survey in the United Kingdom. Mov Disord 2003;18:1139-45.

[11] Hagell P, Nordling S, Reimer J, Grabowski M, Persson U. Resource use and costs in a Swedish cohort of patients with Parkinson's disease. Mov Disord 2002;17:1213-20.

[12] Pressley JC, Louis ED, Tang MX, Cote L, Cohen PD, Glied S, et al. The impact of comorbid disease and injuries on resource use and expenditures in parkinsonism. Neurology 2003;60:87-93.

[13] Chow R, Borean M, Hollenberg D, Merrick J. How aware/knowledgeable are young adults about Parkinson's disease? J Pain Manage 2019; in press.

[14] Chow R, Borean M, Hollenberg D. Awareness of Parkinson's disease: About the survey instrument. J Pain Manage 2019;12(1), in press.

[15] Chow R, Viehweger J, Trasente V, Borean M, Hollenberg D, Lam M, et al. Awareness of Parkinson's disease among young adults in London, Canada. J Pain Manage 2019;12(1), in press.

[16] Ho S, Viehweger J, Trasente V, Ho C, Ng W, Wong M, et al. Awareness of Parkinson's disease among young adults in Toronto, Canada. J Pain Manage 2019;12(1), in press.

[17] Viehweger J, Chow R, Trasente V, Duarte N, Borean M, Hollenberg D, et al. Awareness of Parkinson's disease among young adults in Waterloo, Canada. J Pain Manage 2019;12(1), in press.

[18] Ho S, Viehweger J, Trasente V, Borean M, Hollenberg D, Ferguson T, et al. Awareness of Parkinson's disease among young adults in Halifax, Canada. J Pain Manage 2019;12(1), in press.

[19] Anpalagan T, Chow R, Viehweger J, Trasente V, Borean M, Hollenberg D, et al. Awareness of Parkinson's disease among young adults in Asia. J Pain Manage 2019;12(1), in press.

[20] Viehweger J, Trasente T, Ganguli N, Kang R, Borean M, Hollenberg D, et al. Awareness of Parkinson's disease among young adults in New York State, USA. J Pain Manage 2019;12(1), in press.

[21] Hollenberg D, Viehweger J, Chow R, Rzepka A, Trasente V, Goh S, et al. Awareness of Parkinson's disease among young adults in Dublin, Ireland. J Pain Manage 2019;12(1), in press.

[22] Borean M, Anpalagan T, Trasente V, Midroni L, Midroni C, Hollenberg D, et al. Awareness of Parkinson's disease among young adults in Kingston, Canada. J Pain Manage 2019;12(1), in press.

SECTION FOUR: ACKNOWLEDGMENTS

In: Parkinson's Disease
Editors: Ronald Chow, et al.
ISBN: 978-1-53612-745-4

Chapter 12

ABOUT THE EDITORS

Ronald Chow, BMSc(C), is the Founder and Chair of the Infinitas Research Group, headquartered in London, Ontario, Canada. At the young age of 19 years old, he already has over 170 peer-reviewed publications to his name. He was the recipient of the Ontario Lieutenant Governor's Community Volunteer Award for volunteerism in his community, the Chancellor's Scholarship from Queen's University for excellent academic ability and leadership skills, the George Eastman Young Leaders Award from the University of Rochester for astounding leadership and extensive extracurricular activities, and both the Future of Western Award and Innovation Award from the University of Western Ontario as the most accomplished first-year university student leader in the areas of academics, student government, athletics and philanthropy from Crescent School Email: rchow48@uwo.ca

Jaclyn Viehweger, BMSc(C), is a prominent researcher of Infinitas Research Group. She holds the Gold Duke of Edinburgh Award for her service in the community and commitment to extracurriculars and athletics. Jaclyn graduated from Holy Name of Mary College School in Mississauga having received the Sister Celestine Giertych Social

Justice Award and is now at Western University pursuing a Bachelor of Medical Sciences. Email: jviehweg@uwo.ca

Michael Borean, BMSc(C), Deputy Chair of Infinitas Research Group, has a diverse research background. He has over 45 publications in peer-reviewed journals on topics including oncology, surgery, pharmacy, pediatrics, and public health. During his first year at Western University, Michael won the Innovation Award for leadership and extracurricular involvement. Outside of his research, Michael is heavily involved in student groups for health advocacy, student government, and athletics. He graduated from De La Salle College "Oaklands" in Toronto. Email: mborean@uwo.ca

Drew Hollenberg, BMSc(C), is a Deputy Chair of Infinitas Research Group and a Vice President of the Bicycle Safety and Awareness Club. Also, Drew has published over 55 papers in peer-reviewed journals at 19 years old. He was born in Canada, but soon moved to Tokyo, Japan and then to London, England. Finally returning to Canada again at the age of 14 years, Drew began high school at Crescent School where he won the Graduating Class trophy for outstanding service to the school. Now at Western University, Drew is studying a bachelor in medical sciences. Email: dhollen@uwo.ca

Joav Merrick, MD, MMedSci, DMSc, born and educated in Denmark is professor of pediatrics, child health and human development, Division of Pediatrics, Hadassah Hebrew University Medical Center, Mt Scopus Campus, Jerusalem, Israel and Kentucky Children's Hospital, University of Kentucky, Lexington, Kentucky United States and professor of public health at the Center for Healthy Development, School of Public Health, Georgia State University, Atlanta, United States, the medical director of the Health Services, Division for Intellectual and Developmental Disabilities, Ministry of Social Affairs and Social Services, Jerusalem, the founder and director of the National

Institute of Child Health and Human Development in Israel. Numerous publications in the field of pediatrics, child health and human development, rehabilitation, intellectual disability, disability, health, welfare, abuse, advocacy, quality of life and prevention. Received the Peter Sabroe Child Award for outstanding work on behalf of Danish Children in 1985 and the International LEGO-Prize ("The Children's Nobel Prize") for an extraordinary contribution towards improvement in child welfare and well-being in 1987. Email: jmerrick@zahav.net.il

In: Parkinson's Disease
Editors: Ronald Chow, et al.
ISBN: 978-1-53612-745-4

Chapter 13

ABOUT INFINITAS RESEARCH GROUP, LONDON, ONTARIO, CANADA

Infinitas Research Group (IRG) was founded in 2017, and is currently headquartered in London, Ontario, Canada. Research associates are based around the globe (across Canada, United States, Europe, Asia and Australia), allowing for IRG to conduct research studies on an international scale.

IRG has a special interest in public health issues, and specializes into studying the adolescent and young adult population. IRG has collaborated with many other organizations and has published over 40 papers in its first six months related to topics such as bicycle safety and Alzheimer's disease.

Contact

Ronald Chow
Founder and Chair,
Infinitas Research Group,
London, Ontario, Canada
Email: rchow48@uwo.ca

In: Parkinson's Disease
Editors: Ronald Chow, et al.
ISBN: 978-1-53612-745-4

Chapter 14

About the National Institute of Child Health and Human Development in Israel

The National Institute of Child Health and Human Development (NICHD) in Israel was established in 1998 as a virtual institute under the auspices of the Medical Director, Ministry of Social Affairs and Social Services in order to function as the research arm for the Office of the Medical Director. In 1998 the National Council for Child Health and Pediatrics, Ministry of Health and in 1999 the Director General and Deputy Director General of the Ministry of Health endorsed the establishment of the NICHD.

Mission

The mission of a National Institute for Child Health and Human Development in Israel is to provide an academic focal point for the scholarly interdisciplinary study of child life, health, public health, welfare, disability, rehabilitation, intellectual disability and related aspects of human development. This mission includes research, teaching, clinical work, information and public service activities in the field of child health and human development.

Service and academic activities

Over the years many activities became focused in the south of Israel due to collaboration with various professionals at the Faculty of Health Sciences (FOHS) at the Ben Gurion University of the Negev (BGU). Since 2000 an affiliation with the Zusman Child Development Center at the Pediatric Division of Soroka University Medical Center has resulted in collaboration around the establishment of the Down Syndrome Clinic at that center. In 2002 a full course on "Disability" was established at the Recanati School for Allied Professions in the Community, FOHS, BGU and in 2005 collaboration was started with the Primary Care Unit of the faculty and disability became part of the master of public health course on "Children and society". In the academic year 2005-2006 a one semester course on "Aging with disability" was started as part of the master of science program in gerontology in our collaboration with the Center for Multidisciplinary Research in Aging. In 2010 collaborations with the Division of Pediatrics, Hadassah Hebrew University Medical Center, Jerusalem, Israel around the National Down Syndrome Center and teaching students and residents about intellectual and developmental disabilities as part of their training at this campus.

Research activities

The affiliated staff have over the years published work from projects and research activities in this national and international collaboration. In the year 2000 the International Journal of Adolescent Medicine and

Health and in 2005 the International Journal on Disability and Human Development of De Gruyter Publishing House (Berlin and New York) were affiliated with the National Institute of Child Health and Human Development. From 2008 also the International Journal of Child Health and Human Development (Nova Science, New York), the International Journal of Child and Adolescent Health (Nova Science) and the Journal of Pain Management (Nova Science) affiliated and from 2009 the International Public Health Journal (Nova Science) and Journal of Alternative Medicine Research (Nova Science). All peer-reviewed international journals.

National collaborations

Nationally the NICHD works in collaboration with the Faculty of Health Sciences, Ben Gurion University of the Negev; Department of Physical Therapy, Sackler School of Medicine, Tel Aviv University; Autism Center, Assaf HaRofeh Medical Center; National Rett and PKU Centers at Chaim Sheba Medical Center, Tel HaShomer; Department of Physiotherapy, Haifa University; Department of Education, Bar Ilan University, Ramat Gan, Faculty of Social Sciences and Health Sciences; College of Judea and Samaria in Ariel and in 2011 affiliation with Center for Pediatric Chronic Diseases and National Center for Down Syndrome, Department of Pediatrics, Hadassah Hebrew University Medical Center, Mount Scopus Campus, Jerusalem.

International collaborations

Internationally with the Department of Disability and Human Development, College of Applied Health Sciences, University of Illinois at Chicago; Strong Center for Developmental Disabilities,

Golisano Children's Hospital at Strong, University of Rochester School of Medicine and Dentistry, New York; Centre on Intellectual Disabilities, University of Albany, New York; Centre for Chronic Disease Prevention and Control, Health Canada, Ottawa; Chandler Medical Center and Children's Hospital, Kentucky Children's Hospital, Section of Adolescent Medicine, University of Kentucky, Lexington; Chronic Disease Prevention and Control Research Center, Baylor College of Medicine, Houston, Texas; Division of Neuroscience, Department of Psychiatry, Columbia University, New York; Institute for the Study of Disadvantage and Disability, Atlanta; Center for Autism and Related Disorders, Department Psychiatry, Children's Hospital Boston, Boston; Department of Pediatric and Adolescent Medicine, Western Michigan University Homer Stryker MD School of Medicine, Kalamazoo, Michigan, United States; Department of Paediatrics, Child Health and Adolescent Medicine, Children's Hospital at Westmead, Westmead, Australia; International Centre for the Study of Occupational and Mental Health, Düsseldorf, Germany; Centre for Advanced Studies in Nursing, Department of General Practice and Primary Care, University of Aberdeen, Aberdeen, United Kingdom; Quality of Life Research Center, Copenhagen, Denmark; Nordic School of Public Health, Gottenburg, Sweden, Scandinavian Institute of Quality of Working Life, Oslo, Norway; The Department of Applied Social Sciences (APSS) of The Hong Kong Polytechnic University Hong Kong.

Targets

Our focus is on research, international collaborations, clinical work, teaching and policy in health, disability and human development and to establish the NICHD as a permanent institute in Israel in order to conduct model research and together with the four university schools of public health/medicine in Israel establish a national master and doctoral program in disability and human development at the institute to secure the next generation of professionals working in this often non-prestigious/low-status field of work.

Contact

Joav Merrick, MD, MMedSci, DMSc
Professor of Pediatrics
Medical Director, Health Services, Division for Intellectual and Developmental Disabilities, Ministry of Social Affairs and Social Services, POB 1260, IL-91012 Jerusalem, Israel.
E-mail: jmerrick@zahav.net.il.

In: Parkinson's Disease
Editors: Ronald Chow, et al.
ISBN: 978-1-53612-745-4

Chapter 15

About the Book Series "Disability Studies"

Disability studies is a book series with publications from a multidisciplinary group of researchers, practitioners and clinicians for an international professional forum interested in the broad spectrum of disability, intellectual disability, health and human development.

- Reiter S. Disability from a humanistic perspective: Towards a better quality of life. New York: Nova Science, 2008
- Knotkova H, Cruciani R, Merrick J, eds. Pain. Brain stimulation in the treatment of pain. New York: Nova Science, 2010.
- Prasher VP, ed. Contemporary issues in intellectual disabilities. New York: Nova Science, 2010.
- Lotan M, Merrick J, eds. Rett syndrome: Therapeutic interventions. New York: Nova Science, 2011.
- Satgé D, Merrick J, eds. Cancer in children and adults with intellectual disabilities: Current research aspects. New York: Nova Science, 2011.
- Knotkova H, Cruciani RA, Merrick J, eds. Neural plasticity in chronic pain. New York: Nova Science, 2011.

- Prasher VP. Down syndrome and dementia. A comprehensive and historical review. New York: Nova Science, 2012.
- Merrick J, Aspler S, Morad M, eds. Disability and chronic disease. New York: Nova Science, 2013.
- Tse MMY, Merrick J. Pain and the elderly. New York: Nova Science, 2013.
- Brown RI, Faragher RM, eds. Quality of life and intellectual disability: Knowledge application to other social and educational challenges. New York: Nova Science, 2014.
- Grenon I. From one century to the next: A history of Wrentham State School and the Institutional Model in Massachusetts. New York: Nova Science, 2014.
- Sharkey PM, Merrick J, eds. Virtual reality: People with special needs. New York: Nova Science, 2014.
- Sharkey PM, Merrick J, eds. Virtual reality: Rehabilitation in motor, cognitive and sensorial disorders. New York: Nova Science, 2014.
- Merrick J, Greydanus DE, Patel DR, eds. Intellectual disability: Some current issues New York: Nova Science, 2014.
- Pareto L, Sharkey PM, Merrick J, eds. Technology, rehabilitation and empowerment of people with special needs. New York: Nova Science, 2015.
- Sharkey PM, Merrick J, eds. Recent advances on using virtual reality technologies for rehabilitation. New York: Nova Science, 2016.
- Omar HA, Patel DR, Greydanus DE, Merrick J, eds. Pediatric pain: Current aspects. New York: Nova Science, 2016.
- Palusci VJ, Nazer D, Greydanus DE, Merrick J, eds. Child abuse: Children with disabilities. New York: Nova Science, 2017.
- Powell W, Rizzo A, Sharkey PM, Merrick J, eds. Virtual reality: Recent advances in virtual rehabilitation system design. New York: Nova Science, 2017.
- Powell W, Rizzo A, Sharkey PM, Merrick J, eds. Rehabilitation: Innovations and challenges in the use of virtual reality technologies. New York: Nova Science, 2017.

- Powell W, Sharkey PM, Rizzo A, Merrick J, eds. Virtual reality: Recent advances for health and wellbeing. New York: Nova Science, 2017.

Contact

Professor Joav Merrick, MD, MMedSci, DMSc
Medical Director, Health Services, Division for Intellectual and Developmental Disabilities, Ministry of Social Affairs and Social Services, POBox 1260
IL-91012 Jerusalem, Israel
E-mail: jmerrick@internet-zahav.net

SECTION FIVE: INDEX

INDEX

A

B

C